THE ART OF CONVERSATION
THROUGH SERIOUS ILLNESS

THE ART OF CONVERSATION THROUGH SERIOUS ILLNESS

LESSONS FOR CAREGIVERS

RICHARD P. McQUELLON
MICHAEL A. COWAN

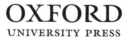

UNIVERSITY PRESS

2010

OXFORD
UNIVERSITY PRESS

Oxford University Press, Inc., publishes works that further
Oxford University's objective of excellence
in research, scholarship, and education.

Oxford   New York
Auckland   Cape Town   Dar es Salaam   Hong Kong   Karachi
Kuala Lumpur   Madrid   Melbourne   Mexico City   Nairobi
New Delhi   Shanghai   Taipei   Toronto

With offices in
Argentina   Austria   Brazil   Chile   Czech Republic   France   Greece
Guatemala   Hungary   Italy   Japan   Poland   Portugal   Singapore
South Korea   Switzerland   Thailand   Turkey   Ukraine   Vietnam

Copyright © 2010 by Oxford University Press

Published by Oxford University Press, Inc.
198 Madison Avenue, New York, New York 10016

www.oup.com

Oxford is a registered trademark of Oxford University Press

Library of Congress Cataloging-in-Publication Data

McQuellon, Richard P., 1949–
The art of conversation through serious illness : lessons for caregivers / Richard P. McQuellon,
Michael A. Cowan.
p.   cm.
Includes bibliographical references and index.
ISBN-13: 978-0-19-538922-7
ISBN-10: 0-19-538922-0
1. Terminal care—Psychological aspects.   2. Death—Psychological aspects.
3. Terminally ill—Psychology.   4. Critically ill—Psychology.
5. Caregivers—Psychology.   I. Cowan, Michael A.   II. Title.
BF789.D4M377 2010
616′.029—dc22
2009034150

1   3   5   7   9   8   6   4   2

Printed in the United States of America
on acid-free paper

To the staff and volunteers of the Cancer Patient Support Program
Comprehensive Cancer Center
Wake Forest University Baptist Medical Center
Winston-Salem, North Carolina
To our mothers: Kathleen McQuellon and Marie Cowan
To our wives: Cyndee and Kathleen
To our children: Meghan, Brendan, Kristin, Katrin,
Mairin, Kendall, and Rebecca
To our patients: They taught us how to walk together with courage
in mortal time.

CONTENTS

Acknowledgments xi

Prologue xv

INTRODUCTION 3

The Birth of Possibility 3

Living with Mortality 5

Guidance for Caregivers in Mortal Time 8

PART I

THE MANY MEANINGS OF MORTAL TIME 13

Mortal Time: How Long Does It Last? 14

The Multiple Meanings of Mortal Time 16

Shattered Assumptions 18

Creating Meaning 19

Coping Styles 20

What to Expect in Mortal Time 24

The Challenge and the Invitation of Mortal Time 33

A Question of Balance 34

The Prospect of Despair 35

Finding Meaning 37

Living in Mortal Time 41

Sources of Hope 44

Nevertheless, There Is Meaning 45

Part II

Hope from Conversation 49

Hope for the Day 49

Avoiding Gloom 52

False Hope 53

Conversation 54

Healing Conversation: Basic Elements 56

Talking In and About Mortal Time 59

Conversation Partners 62

Empathy 64

Becoming Properly Empathetic 66

Receiving Empathy 68

Honesty: What Can I Say? 70

The Right Words 72

Acknowledging Fear 73

Everyday Conversation with Friends 75

Platitudes:

Let's Hope for the Best and Prepare for the Worst 77

You First! 80

The Humane Use of Words:

Effective Phrases in Mortal Time 81

Consideration and Disciplined Spontaneity 82

Censored Conversation vs. Active Listening 85

How Much Time Do I Have? 87

Appreciating Everyday Chatter 88

Denial? 89

Healthy Conversation About Dying   92
Practical Conversation   94

PART III

GUIDANCE FOR CAREGIVERS   99

Being a Companion in Mortal Time   99
Kind Companions   100
The Costs and Risks of Companionship   104
The Nine Personal Virtues Most
Needed in Mortal Time   106
A Word to Caregivers   117
Resilience and Absorbing Suffering   118
Empathy Shift   120
Sharing the Darkness   122
Mending   123
The Art of Conversation Through Serious Illness   123

Notes   125
Bibliography   131
Index   135
Author Contact Information   144

ACKNOWLEDGMENTS

The Psychosocial Oncology (POP) and Cancer Patient Support Programs (CPSP) at Wake Forest University Baptist Medical Center have provided our stage for encountering the serious illness of cancer. Both programs are designed to reduce the suffering of cancer patients and their family members during the diagnostic, treatment, and survivorship process. The CPSP consists of six staff members, approximately 30 weekly volunteers, and more than 100 community volunteers who give of themselves tirelessly. Marian Douglas, Ann Hanes, Kathy Janeway, Agnes Berry, Skip Boyles, Carolyn Ferree, Glen Lesser, Susan Kennedy, and all the members of the CPSP

Advisory Committee have given through the years so that patients may benefit. We are thankful to all of our volunteers and especially to Dr. Eddie Easley for his courage, grace, and careful reading of an early draft of this text. He and Roger Jordan are on duty each week comforting patients and family members in our comprehensive cancer center. They know, firsthand, what it means to manage serious illness.

We are honored to work alongside the nurses, physicians, physician's assistants, chaplains, social workers, counselors, and other health-care professionals who strive to reduce suffering and promote healing each and every day. We especially thank Hy Muss for his generous spirit and Bayard Powell, David Hurd, Julia Cruz, Suzanne Carroll, Frank Torti, Ed Shaw, William Blackstock, Ed Levine, Jennie Morris, Pat Johnson, and Maureen Sintich for their leadership efforts in our Comprehensive Cancer Center.

We are indebted to a number of our friends, students, and colleagues who have contributed to this book in many ways including reading earlier drafts and offering useful comments. Richard Chiles, Cyndee McQuellon, Kathy and Jerry McShane, Cassie Campbell, Katie Duckworth, Tony Miller, Patrick Ober, Tom Dubose, Bill Applegate, Sue Stewart, Anne Kissel, Barry Maine, Paul Savage, Gail Hurt,

Will Voelzke, Daniel Burke, Jared Rejeski, Weston Saunders, Randy Beard, Linda Gitter, Loretta Muss, Wilson Somerville, and Vernon Foster all provided helpful and encouraging feedback. On our watch, hundreds of people over the years have entered the chaotic world of serious illness with grace and courage. We thank them all and the following for showing us the way: Dennis and Sandy O'Hara, Nel Martin, Patrice Radke, Lynn Felder, Ray Joyner, Kathleen and Robert Niles, Bill and Linda Garwood, Dave and Peggy Slater and Pam and Mark Rabil.

Anne Adkins, a CPSP volunteer, gave us vision and encouragement. The students of the course "Living in Mortal Time: Clinical and Literary Perspectives" at Wake Forest University gave valuable feedback on the text. The Shades of Praise Interracial choir of New Orleans inspires us. Philadelphia Jesuit Volunteer Corp members Andrew Keating, Brendan McQuellon, John Thompson, Mary Niehaus, Mo Patterson, and Shalani Thomas give us hope. Fr. Conall McHugh, OFM Conv., consistently provided encouragement with a simple question: "How's the book coming?" Canice Connors, OFM Conv., helped by asking, "Where are you called?" The community of Franciscan friars and Sisters of St. Francis, Philadelphia provide daily sustenance for the soul working with serious illness.

Finally, we thank the following for supporting this project: The Herbert and Ann Brenner Fund; The Kathryn A. Millward Fund; The Barbara D. Smitherman Memorial Trust; The Bertha Long CPSP Fund; The Higgenbotham Memorial CPSP Fund, the Belk-Glenn Fund for Cancer Patients, The Kulynych Family Foundation, The Lacey Foundation, and the Jane Hanes Memorial Fund. Their foresight and generosity gave us the time and resources to write and produce this book.

RPM

MAC

PROLOGUE

On Earth[1]
by Franz Wright

Resurrection of the little apple tree outside
my window, leaf-
light of late
in the April
called her eyes, forget
forget –
but how
How does one go about dying?
Who on earth
is going to teach me –
The world
is filled with people
who have never died

THE ART OF CONVERSATION
THROUGH SERIOUS ILLNESS

INTRODUCTION[1]

THE BIRTH OF POSSIBILITY

A profound but rarely considered reality is that the moment of our birth promises the inevitability of our death. We enter mortal time when we are born. Youth with its promise rarely considers this, while the elderly may be all too aware of it. In this book we will consider the experience of facing life-threatening illness, when the prospect of ending becomes all too real. At one extreme, mortality can be trivialized by offhand comments like, "We all have to go sometime." At the other, it can provoke morbid preoccupation. In these pages, we will navigate between the extremes of obliviousness and obsession, providing guidance for those who would be engaged companions in mortal time. Below, Mary's story illustrates the complex forces that come to bear on a particular encounter with mortality, when illness appears incurable.

When Mary's physician told her that her breast cancer had returned and spread to her lungs and liver, her calm reaction took him by surprise. The young physician in training felt that Mary didn't understand the seriousness of her predicament. When I spoke with Mary in consultation, she was sitting at the bedside in some discomfort but managing her pain reasonably well. She understood that her cancer had now moved to her liver and lungs and that it was not curable. She said that her main physician was "the man upstairs," but she also believed that "God works through people like you and the doctors and nurses." She further stated that she trusted her doctors and relied on their input. However, she was in the hands of God, who would be the ultimate physician in her case. She was dignified, humble, and unafraid of talking about what might lie ahead for her. She had buried her father and cared for a brother disabled by a stroke within the past year. She had grown familiar with the possibility of dying. Her caring physician was not critical of her, but puzzled by what seemed to be her "denial" of her situation. She was prepared to discuss the limits to her life, yet hopeful that she would be touched with a miracle. For her this was not denial but rather a deep faith in the future, whatever it held.

Mary was calm in the face of her diagnosis, her physician was puzzled by her response to life-threatening information, and the consulting caregiver was struck by their differing responses. This incident highlights the power of death's multiple meanings to shape feelings and behavior. While only one person in this story faces grave illness, all three—the patient, her physician, and the consultant—are facing the reality of living with death's possibility. Mortality has a different meaning for each of them, as it does for everyone it touches. These meanings color how people feel, think, and communicate as they turn to face mortality together.

LIVING WITH MORTALITY

This book is about living gracefully with the possibility of death, whether it is on the doorstep or in the unforeseeable future. We are professional caregivers, but we have written this book with a particular concern for friends and family who are accompanying loved ones during the diagnosis and treatment of a life-threatening, life-changing illness such as cancer. We use the phrase "mortal time" more to capture the experience of being acutely aware of one's own mortality than to describe a particular period. While we all are set into mortal time from birth, illness can call mortality into sharp focus. We use the term "life threatening" in these pages to refer to situations where a person believes that his illness could shorten his natural lifespan in the immediate or more distant future.

Receiving a life-threatening diagnosis can be profoundly disturbing. Author Michael Lerner has likened receiving a cancer diagnosis to being dropped into a jungle with no survival skills or tools.[2] Often without warning, the patient, family, and friends find themselves on alien, anxiety-provoking ground. Here we provide map and compass for those facing death directly or as companions of loved ones facing territory that is inherently frightening. We offer reflections on the momentous rite of passage that we call "mortal time" through real-life stories and possible answers to questions that people may have when moving into mortal time. We consider how one can listen carefully and respond thoughtfully when facing life-threatening illness.

Our purpose in writing this book is to encourage frank, life-affirming conversation for those facing the prospect of death. We offer a philosophy of "how to be" in mortal time rather than a prescription for "what to do" there, although we do offer concrete suggestions for conversation. Death is not unspeakable and need not be avoided until the "last minute," when a precious life is ebbing quickly, and opportunities for dialogue may be dramatically limited. In fact, embracing mortality honestly and compassionately can open the hearts of family members, friends, and other caregivers to speak of life in all its richness and promise. These conversations call for sensitivity and courage.

Dying is part of living and needs to be "talkable." In the American culture famous for collective denial of death, this means going against the grain. We do not advocate morbid preoccupation with death, nor pushing the "death talk," but rather courageous acknowledgment and honest, sensitive engagement with a central fact of life: all of our lives are time-limited. Mortal time is only a reminder of that challenging, difficult truth, which each of us faces, more or less consciously, throughout life. For the professional caregiver, mortal time may be a daily companion; for the rest of us, opportunities to befriend mortality will appear unpredictably over the course of our lifetimes.

GUIDANCE FOR CAREGIVERS
IN MORTAL TIME

What you will read here is drawn from more than 20 years of intense experience with patients and their caregivers in a comprehensive cancer center as well as personal encounters with serious illness and dying. In the field of cancer treatment, the term "caregiver" is often used to describe family members who have a major part in assisting a relative diagnosed with some form of cancer. We broaden that meaning to include professionals, friends, and non-family members such as hospital and hospice volunteers, who are involved in the care of patients facing serious illness. Our primary audience is the person who would be a companion to anyone in mortal time.

In Part I: "The Many Meanings of Mortal Time," we consider the personal experience of patients and caregivers confronting life-threatening diagnoses, and focus on the role of meaning in that confrontation. This section lays the groundwork for addressing the main question of the book, which appears in Part II: "Hope from Conversation," namely, how can caregivers walk with compassion and honesty in the inevitably disturbing company of mortality? In Part III: "Guidance for Caregivers," we focus our attention on being companions to others in mortal time. We close with a word to caregivers about the hazards and blessings of mortal time. Given the intense emotions that arise in the face of death, it is hard to think clearly and reflect wisely when its prospect looms closely.

Even though the approach you will find in these pages emerged from direct experience with patients and caregivers contending with the diagnosis and treatment of cancer, it is applicable to anyone facing life-threatening circumstances. We have changed the names of all patients whose stories we share, remaining true to their stories while protecting their anonymity. Our hope is that people facing mortality, those who love them, and those who care for them will find in these pages compassion for their suffering, the consolation of meaning, and practical guidance for the challenging journey through mortal time, which awaits us all.

PART I

THE MANY MEANINGS OF
MORTAL TIME

*"In a dark time, the eye begins to see, I meet my shadow in
the deepening shade."*[1]
–THEODORE ROETHKE

n our work, we use "mortal time" to mean the experience
of human beings confronting the prospect of death.[2]
This confrontation can stimulate intense feelings, a flurry
of thoughts, and erratic or unusual behavior. In the
broadest sense, mortal time is entered whenever death
comes near, and that can happen either directly or vicariously. Hearing the words "you have cancer," signing a
medical consent form where death is a possible medical
"complication," or momentarily losing control of a car on
an icy street are direct and acute experiences of mortal time.
Learning of a loved one's cancer diagnosis, losing a family
member in an automobile accident, or reading about a child
gone missing are vicarious experiences of mortal time.

As we noted in our introduction, the focus in this book is on the particular and powerful experience of entering mortal time when someone receives a diagnosis of life-threatening illness. It may be an illness where a rapid progression toward death is looming, or where there is only the distant possibility that death will be caused by the illness.

MORTAL TIME:
HOW LONG DOES IT LAST?

There are, of course, many instances in which people far exceed their statistically predicted life span. This holds true whether it be the prediction of a physician in the midst of treating an illness or the projected life span of an insurance life-expectancy table.[3]

When mortal time is entered with the diagnosis of a serious illness, it may stretch from days to years, with patients encountering both helpful treatments that lead to periods of remission and recurrences of disease requiring additional treatment. Some of the chronically ill may never experience a time when it is apparent that they are dying. The interval between living and dying that we are concerned with here is not chronological time, measured in days, weeks, and months. The hallmark of mortal time is the person's unique biological, psychological, social, and spiritual experience of the prospect and meaning of death, a prospect that confronts their caregivers as well. Mortal time is "kairos" time, the ancient Greek word meaning the time of decisions.[4] When someone enters mortal time directly, their caregivers enter the same "time zone" vicariously. How they speak and what they do in mortal time together affects the quality and meaning of life for all involved, in the moment and beyond.

When Mary, whom you met earlier, was told by her physician about the return and spread of her cancer, both of them entered mortal time, one directly, the other vicariously. The diagnosis of a likely terminal illness abruptly and intensely brings home the reality of death to those involved. When such an illness is diagnosed, all those it touches are thrown into mortal time. This stark meeting with mortality boils down to two inevitably disturbing realities: someone is facing the prospect of death, and those involved know it.

Ironically, we have heard people in mortal time describe the puzzlement they sometimes see on the faces of those who observe that they are still alive in spite of the predictions of death. Their faces seem to say: "Are you still alive? I thought you were supposed to die." We have seen a version

of this very awkward conversation unfold between professional caregivers and their patients. And we have listened
to people say how awkward it is when their mortal time zone
extends far beyond its predicted course. After all, how is one
to act with those who are "supposed to be dead"? Indeed, for
many of us, there is an unspoken assumption about how long
one can linger on the doorstep of death, an expectation that
remains unclear until the prospect of demise come into focus,
which happens only when the meaning of a cancer diagnosis
is fully understood.

The Multiple Meanings of Mortal Time

What are the possible meanings of a direct or vicarious
confrontation with mortality? Patients and their caregivers
encounter the imminent prospect of death as they do other
life events, through the looking glass of their own personal
history. Psychotherapist Jerome Frank called the unique
perspective that each person brings to life situations the
"assumptive world."[5] Think of your assumptive world as
the story you have personally gleaned from living, your
personal account of what life means and your role within
it. That story is the meaning you give the events of your life,
birthplace, schooling, vocation, etc. For example, a person
growing up in a spiritual tradition emphasizing life after

death may believe (assume) that death is the midwife to another world. The assumption is that some form of life goes on after the body dies. Carrying this assumption into mortal time will give that time meaning that will be different from the person who believes that the end of the body means the end of the person.

The overall story and the specific assumptions that guide people in everyday life and, in particular, in mortal time are continually updated. Each person's story makes possible and yet limits his understanding and interpretation of events. Those interpretations in turn make possible and limit how he feels and acts in all of life's circumstances, including death. For example, a first-born daughter of working parents with a mother on second shift would likely be thrust into a caregiver role early, as she regularly looks after her younger siblings in the parents' absence. Her assumptive world or life story would likely have a very strong "taking care of others" component. These assumptions operate automatically, often as "shoulds," in this case as, "I should always be responsible for my brothers and sisters." This view would contrast with that of one who was the youngest of six, the "baby" of the family, always being taken care of by others as she was growing up. We all carry personal assumptive worlds, the product of our life experience and inherited capabilities. Assumptive worlds are both stable and changeable over time.

Mary held a strong belief that God cares and would continue to care for her. She had faith in the future even when cancer returned to shorten her life. This belief was the anchor of her assumptive world. She appeared to her physician to be unrealistic; he thought that she was not fully aware of her situation. His assumptive world did not include faith in a spiritual being. Hers did. From his vantage point, she was in denial. From the consultant's perspective, Mary was not only able to comprehend the seriousness of her illness but empowered to face it by her conviction that she was in the hands of a power higher than medicine. People deal with the inevitable trauma of entering mortal time differently, depending on what they bring to it, especially their differing assumptive worlds. The personal assumptions of patients and caregivers shape their entire experience of mortal time.

SHATTERED ASSUMPTIONS

Personal assumptions can be radically altered in an instant. As psychologist Ronnie Janoff-Bulman noted, "shattered assumptions" can occur when any major crisis calls into question three universal, but usually implicit, assumptions that we all make: the world is benevolent, the world is meaningful, and we are worthy.[6] The diagnosis of a life-threatening illness like cancer can cast these assumptions into doubt and even "shatter them to pieces." The benevolence and meaningfulness of the world can be quickly called into question when death comes calling in the form of cancer. This confrontation can lead to heightened anxiety and the lament "Why me?" as the illusion that we are immune to death is confronted first hand. How we adjust after our assumptions are shaken depends on whether we despair or remain hopeful upon entering mortal time. How does hope survive shattered assumptions? How is meaning restored in a newly determined time-limited world, a world of mortal time?

CREATING MEANING

In order to appreciate the meaning that can be drawn from life-changing experiences, it is useful to consider how meaning is created. One classic view is that the meaning of something resides within it. Another is that the meaning of something is in the mind of the interpreter. We take a third position: Meaning happens "in between," when an event and its interpreter meet. We don't feel, think, and act the way we do solely because something happens, but also because of what it *means* to us. In mortal time, patients and caregivers meet the prospect of death, and what that meeting will be like depends both on what it brings to us and what we bring to it. What we bring is our own assumptive world, which could include many experiences with life-threatening illness and death or none at all. The person with no experience in mortal time may find the first encounter a meaning-shattering experience and very difficult to cope with. Indeed, an entire nation can be forced into a new understanding of mortality when confronting death on an unprecedented scale, as the United States did during the Civil War.[7]

Coping Styles

Psychologist David Cella has described four styles of coping with cancer that reflect different assumptive worlds: realists, opportunists, zealots, and fighters.[8] These styles may be thought of as ways of interpreting and acting when faced with a life-threatening situation. Each style of coping represents one way that a person can respond to entry into mortal time, but this list is by no means exhaustive or exclusive. Many people combine two or more of these coping styles. Even though they were created with

‘

cancer in mind, they can serve for other types of illness as well, e.g., chronic obstructive pulmonary disease or congestive heart failure. We have modified the definition of his categories and have added one other.

Realists understand that the odds are against them. Cella describes them as people who see little hope in their situation. We think of realists as those who can tolerate the prospect of death without sinking into despair. A realist would perhaps see a different kind of hope emerging from mortal time, such as the hope of a life hereafter. Mary, who was facing incurable breast cancer, spoke of this reality. Her hope was not for cure but acceptance of the progression of disease made tolerable by her faith in life after death.

People who see no hope in their situation we would call pessimists. *Pessimists* have a tendency to stress the negative or unfavorable or to take the gloomiest possible view of a situation. They see the glass as half empty. Whatever wrong that can happen will happen. They are likely to consider any optimistic statement as "false hope," rather than seeing a range of possibilities in their illness from good treatment options to the real possibility of rapid decline and death. In the pages to come you will meet Thomas, a young man who speaks pessimistically of his impending death even while considering treatment options. A pessimistic outlook can lead to despair.

Opportunists would like to reduce the daily stress that accompanies treatment and the awareness of one's fatal illness; however, they are not willing to expend the energy it takes to do so. An opportunist is someone who takes advantage of an opportunity to achieve an end, in this case cure of their disease, often with little regard for consequences. They may simply wait for those around them to provide the right opportunities for cure or help. Then they will take advantage of the situation. They may be passive in their approach to their own medical care.

Zealots think that the mind has the power to heal the body. They may believe that "love, medicine, and miracles" are all that are needed for sure cure, and perhaps conventional medicine may not be needed either. Their frenetic activity and intensity may help relieve the natural anxiety that comes with suffering and the possibility of death. Some zealots would rather pursue one more unusual avenue than contemplate the prospect of their own death. They are likely to be saying, "I am going to beat this cancer no matter what" even while their body is being overwhelmed by disease. Their strong convictions and often unconventional beliefs can make professional caregivers uncomfortable. For example, they may enthusiastically embrace non-medical therapies such as herbal preparations and colon cleansing to the exclusion of conventional, accepted approaches like chemotherapy. This perspective can often rob a family of the comfort of embracing their loved one in the deep mutual care that can emerge in the shadow of death. Final blessings can be forever missed while someone flees mortal time pursuing a miracle cure in a distant country.

On the positive side, zealots can energize those around them and create positive energy in the early stages of life-threatening illness, when the illness trajectory is ambiguous. They do this with a dogged determination and an unrelenting pursuit of cure even when it is impossible.

Fighters are adaptive copers. Like zealots, they believe in the power of the mind to influence the body. However, they are fully aware of their mortality and have the ability to take advantage of useful messages and information from the popular press, research, or their professional caregivers, rather than investing all hope in radical, unorthodox treatments. They tend to gravitate toward more proven treatments and approaches that are under development within conventional medical care, e.g., medications that are experimental. Fighters generally cope well by adopting an adaptive, upbeat attitude as well as developing a factual understanding of the powerful biology of cancer.

As an alternative to the metaphor of "fighting" life-threatening illness, author Carol Orsborn has suggested a sixth type of coper—*peacemakers*—those who follow the ways of letting go and relaxing deeply in response to serious illness, especially cancer.[9]

One patient told us that she didn't fit any of these labels neatly, but was a blend of realist and fighter, paying close attention to the facts of her disease but never giving up on treatment possibilities. Because they bring such different assumptions to life-threatening illness, realists, pessimists, opportunists, zealots, fighters, and peacemakers experience mortal time quite differently as patients and caregivers. It would be true to say not just that each faces mortal time differently, but that each faces a different reality in mortal time.

What to Expect in Mortal Time

While patients bring diverse assumptions, feelings, and coping styles into mortal time, four common experiences await almost everyone who arrives there.

First, entry into mortal time is profoundly disturbing. *When Dustin began having trouble swallowing, he assumed it was a symptom that would pass. When it persisted and became worse he* saw his family physician, who sent him to a gastroenterologist. An endoscopy and biopsy revealed cancer of the esophagus. The diagnosis shocked and frightened him, catapulting him into mortal time abruptly and painfully. He had found out that this was a difficult cancer to treat successfully. He called to discuss what was happening prior to talking with his surgeon and oncologist about a treatment plan. He was understandably deeply distressed and on the verge of tears during our conversation. He apologized for his raw emotion, easily triggered. "I'm sorry. These tears just seem to come in waves. I don't have much control. This has never happened before. I'm not at work today; I'm out shopping for a car with my son. That helps to keep my mind off it." He went on to say that he was working with his doctors to get a treatment plan in place while contending with intrusive thoughts about the prospect of not seeing his children grow into adults.

What was most disturbing to Dustin? —the potential loss of a hoped-for future. He might not ever see his daughter marry or his hoped-for grandchildren enter the world.

Dustin was coping by deeply experiencing the painful, shocking reality of his diagnosis, absorbing the prospect of loss while bravely carrying on being a good father. He was fortunate to have a loving, sensitive spouse. His family members were in shock too, as they learned just what such a diagnosis implied for the near future. They could not help but wonder just how long the future of their family unit would last. The diagnosis of esophageal cancer tested them and brought new awareness into a courageous, caring family.

Absorbing the shock of diagnosis is difficult enough, but the language of health-care providers and others can force people into mortal time harshly. Statements such as "Only 15–20% of people with your stage of lung cancer survive five years or more," delivered matter-of-factly, are stunning to someone unaccustomed to the statistical language of medicine. It can be especially painful if followed by, "If I were you, I would get my affairs in order." Such comments may suggest gross insensitivity or tactlessness on the part of medical providers. While this may be the case, the reality is often more complex. Patients often elicit blunt statements by demanding that health-care providers "be straight with me" or "give me some kind of time frame." One of our patients was highly distressed when her physician called her on the phone and said, "You have colon cancer and need surgery immediately." She described him as curt, short, and "uncaring." It was his manner that disturbed her the most. The physician making this phone call may have been simply attempting to convey the gravity of her situation in order to encourage her to move quickly.

We aren't blaming either party, but are simply pointing out the complexity of communication in such intense situations, and how easily it can go wrong. Even when the diagnosis of a life-threatening illness goes well and is conveyed with care, it can be stunning, even shocking, to its direct and vicarious recipients.

It is senseless to look for fault with caregivers and patients, who may fail to communicate well in these trying conversations. Both are attempting to talk about a nearly incomprehensible event, that is, the prospect of death for a human being. Professional caregivers and patients, however, do not enter these exchanges as equals. The former are not superhuman, but are rightfully expected to assume greater responsibility for how the conversation proceeds because of their training and experience. Fortunately, medical educators are ever more aware of the necessity of giving their students some training in respectful, compassionate communication when entering conversations in mortal time.[10]

A second common experience in mortal time is preoccupation with the prospect of death. The statement "People with your disease usually have about six months to live" is stark and terrifying. It can set off a cascade of worries and near-constant rumination about the illness, financial concerns, tearful episodes about the anticipated future, and intense anxiety about what might happen to children. Fortunately, people cannot think about imminent death constantly over a long period of time. To keep the prospect of death in the forefront of one's mind continuously robs the present of hopeful, life-affirming activity. This results in a form of "the feared future dominating the lived present." A total focus on dying is impossible because the mundane tasks of living—working, eating, dressing, sleeping, and so on— will invariably interrupt even the most intense preoccupations. Nevertheless, intrusive thoughts, such as the type Dustin experienced, are common during first entry into mortal time. Dustin was helped by tending to the task of looking for a car for his son, directing attention outside his own worries.

The focus of patients and caregivers on endings and what the end means will shift from foreground to background over a period of moments, hours, days, weeks, months, even years. This fluctuation depends upon many things, including the frequency of ongoing medical tests, medical news regarding the success of treatment, the occurrence or recurrence of symptoms, the patient's own understanding of progress in the development of new healing treatments for his or her condition, and the responses of other people to his or her condition. The uniquely personal experience of mortal time is a constantly changing kaleidoscope of fears, fantasies, and worries, including the waxing and waning of hope for the future.

Considering one's mortality may be more or less useful for planning purposes for things such as life or health insurance. It would not be unusual for a 75-year-old to be contemplating final things; however, we would be surprised if a teenager was caught up in thoughts about death for long periods. There are times during the life cycle when thinking about mortality would be likely to occur.

A third common experience when people encounter mortal time is a shocking sense of loss. Life's formerly taken-for-granted possibilities are shaken by the prospect of death. These losses include every aspect of life—family, friends, career, interests, and commitments—including, at the deepest level, the loss of self, the end of "me." In one disruptive instant, the hopes and dreams on my horizon are called into question. The unspoken assumption that "life will go on" has been snatched away in one terrible moment and transformed into "life will go on without me." An inevitable but unexpected ending has suddenly come into sight, transforming everything that stretches between now and it. People feel and express this sense of loss at the prospect of death in widely varying forms, depending, once again, on the assumptions they bring to it. One may expect to find nothing beyond this life or, as one patient said, "When I am gone, that is it, nothingness, blackness, the end." Another may see death as the transformation of herself into a transcendent being with eternal life in the hereafter.

Loss permeates the life span so much that it is a normal part of natural growth and development, but the introduction into mortality may be totally unexpected and new for a younger person with little history of loss or a common experience for an 80-year-old familiar with the death of loved ones. It might be thought of as the "grief" that accompanies human development. That is, as we progress through normal developmental stages of life from birth to death, we naturally experience loss, loss of physical and mental abilities, loss of family and friends to death, and the loss of our children from the home as they grow up and move on.

The loss of valued roles that individuals play in their families is a common and disturbing occurrence in mortal time. When a life-threatening diagnosis is announced, it will likely be accompanied by rigorous treatment. In cancer medicine, surgery, radiation therapy, or chemotherapy portend major role changes that may cause permanent or temporary changes in daily functioning. Below you will see that Jim learned it was devastating to lose the ability to take part in the little things that make up daily life. It was just as hard to be forced to watch his wife struggle to take on his former responsibilities in addition to her own.

Jim was hospitalized for five weeks for initial treatment of acute leukemia. This meant that he had to take temporary medical leave from his work as a high school teacher and could see his two young sons only on the weekends during treatment. Furthermore, he developed an infection midway through his treatment, requiring isolation and no visits from his children. His two most highly valued roles of teacher and father were temporarily lost. He commented, "What I really miss is wrestling with them on the living room floor." At the same time, his wife Terri had to assume his role on top of her own, managing the household and tending to the children while maintaining her job as a medical social worker. Her caregiver role was very demanding over the course of hospitalization, as the entire family had to adjust to their changing roles.

Finally, no one returns unchanged from a confrontation with death. The changes may be dramatic, taking surprising, even liberating, twists.

"My cancer was a gift to me."
When Joyce said this, her consultant was puzzled. She went on to say that once she had gotten over the initial treatment and

reconsidered the nature of her life, she knew that some things had to change. She saw that she was living in a rut. Her life consisted of working eight plus hours a day and coming home to cook, clean, and manage all the household chores. With new resolve and energy, she told her husband that things were going to be different. She now saw that her life span may be shortened. Even though treatment was proceeding well, and she had an excellent prognosis, her brush with the possibility of death had changed her forever. "I'm just not going to do that anymore. I'm not going to work full time and do everything at home. The chores are going to be shared or else. This is a whole new life for me."

These words come from a woman who had not spoken up in her marriage for many years. They convey the sense of urgency that mortal time brings to some, the urge to deal with things differently, to make important changes. Precious life is waning, and it's time to act. Joyce found new and liberating possibilities awaiting her in mortal time. One of the consequences, of course, is that loved ones and others will have to change also, as relationships find a new balance. A life-threatening diagnosis for one person means changes for everyone in that person's web of relationships. Joyce's cancer diagnosis caused her to examine her most important relationship, her marriage.

Unexpectedly, hope for a better life arose from seeing her marriage through the lens of life-threatening illness, giving her a different perspective. Mortal time has its own graces.

How we experience oncoming death depends largely on what we bring to it. How mortal time feels and what we can do within it depends on what it means to us.

The Challenge and the Invitation of Mortal Time
Human beings live with three fundamental questions, the same ones that give rise to the great fruits of culture—religion, philosophy, literature, music, and art:

- Where did I come from?
- What is my purpose?
- What is my destiny?

Such profound questions rarely emerge in daily life. Weeks, months, years, even a lifetime can slip away without a serious brush with them. But particular life events—birth, a close call in an accident, serious illness, or unexpected blessings—have a way of bringing them up, inviting at least a moment of reflection in passing. Ever since human beings emerged within the cosmos some 200,000 years ago, one life event above all others—our impending death or that of a loved one—has been the prime provoker of meaning-of-life questions. The questions of origin, purpose, and destiny invite deep reflection with no guarantees. People find different answers; some are liberated, and some burdened. The question of purpose—what am I doing? for what reason?—is an especially powerful motivator. We focus primarily on the issue of purpose and meaning in the next section.

A Question of Balance

Anna Ornstein, a survivor of Auschwitz, has written eloquently of how we human beings always live in the balance of hope and despair.[11] The source of hope is meaning; the source of despair is meaninglessness. Most of us continue on our way from day to day because we find enough value and significance in our daily work, family, and civic life to keep us going. When meaning sags a little, we find ourselves asking, "Is this all there is?" Depression intensifies such questions, and can undermine meaning radically, pushing us toward the abyss of despair. Past a certain point, despair can move human beings to its logical consequence—suicide. It is no accident that cancer patients have twice the suicide rate as the general population. Absent hope, life is literally unsustainable.

The everyday hope and purpose that keep us going are interrupted by the possibility of impending death. Those who find themselves in mortal time and the ones who care for them are vulnerable to despair. For some, the balance of hope and despair is precarious. Professional caregivers often err on the side of presenting the worst case; they fear raising too much hope for patients when the disease outcome is likely death. The ethical obligation of professional caregivers is to present to patients diagnosed with life-threatening conditions a picture of their situation based on accurate medical knowledge. This casts patients and professionals into very challenging conversations. What is a physician to say to a patient who asks, "How long do I have to live? I want to see my grandchildren grow up." Would it be giving false hope to say, "Let's do the best we can" to a man with advanced cancer with an expected life span of six to twelve months? We discuss the idea of "false hope" in more depth in Part II.

The Prospect of Despair

"I am a dead man." Thomas, a 19-year-old college student who had recently completed chemotherapy for acute leukemia, shocked a

seasoned professional caregiver with these words. They were spoken during a bedside meeting right after Thomas had learned that the treatment had failed and he was now to prepare to undergo bone marrow transplantation. He understood the poor odds of this procedure for him and was in despair about the chance of cure. His powerful words stunned the consultant, even after nearly twenty years of dramatic encounters with cancer patients. What does one say to a young man who makes what might be fairly characterized as a realistic and truthful assessment of his situation? It was difficult to respond beyond an initial nod in recognition of his plight. After all, platitudes aside, what is one to say in the face of authentic despair? What motivates a person to describe himself as "a dead man" in the presence of others? And how does a caregiver respond to such intense communication?

In mortal time, we acutely feel the anxiety and vulnerability of the balance between extended life and impending death and may well find ourselves tipping toward despair momentarily or for extended periods. What is it that threatens the meaning of life itself? A great student of the human condition, Clifford Geertz, offers this answer: too much complexity, too much evil, or too much pain.[12] "Too much" simply means more than we can bear. In mortal time, our own pain or that of those we love can become more than we feel we can bear. The emotional signal that we are approaching the limit of bearability is the tug of despair, calling into question our ordinary lives and agendas, raising the fundamental questions of meaning, draining away our resolve and energy. Here, in mortal time, those questions face us not as academic exercises or voluntary personal growth activities, but in all their high-voltage, anxious, existential, spiritual power.

"I am a dead man." Thomas was acutely experiencing what we call mortal time, realizing that death is near, in this case, even in the inner sanctum of high-tech medicine. This self-pronounced death sentence reveals a young man's agony on the terrain of despair and issues a stark, angry challenge to any caregiver daring to engage him on that terrible ground. They are words of revelation and invitation, of disclosure and challenge. They give us a precious, painful glimpse of how harrowing the course of mortal time can be. For Thomas, the balance between hope and despair had tipped in favor of dark rumination and hopelessness.

Finding Meaning

However, mortal time is not merely a frightening event that we must cope with periodically, but also one with the power to enhance life by flooding it with meaning. The diagnosis of life-threatening illness can bear the gift of intense and precious opportunities to reaffirm cherished meanings and discover new ones. How so? Martin Heidegger offered twentieth-century philosophy's most influential account of the character and significance of death.[13] His penetrating insight was that death is not primarily a biological event facing us at some as-yet-undetermined future point; rather, it is both a personal confrontation with the time limits of our existence and the most powerful and challenging invitation to live the time we have as fully and truly as possible. Heidegger realized that the limit named "death" sets the boundary of our very existence. The fundamental psychological and spiritual demand facing mortal human beings is accepting that our lives are limited. Embracing the fact that we will die can propel us into living authentically. Failing to confront the fact of our finitude, that our lifetimes and possibilities are not endless, leaves us scattered, unfocused, and prey to the unending procession of cultural fads and addictions. Time "gets away" from us, and we realize too late that cherished hopes for ourselves, our families, and our communities will go unrealized. Facing the truth of Augustine's famous words: "When we finally lay down, we lay down for a long time," without succumbing to despair, demoralization, and paralysis, has a unique power to focus our attention and energize our living.[14] Acknowledging fully that our life story will end can propel us into living it more fully and richly. Turning and facing the fact that we will die, so that we may live more fully, is the paradoxical promise of mortal time and perhaps its most profound source of hope.

Resolutely examining one's life in the face of death can lead to more meaningful and life-giving forms of thinking, feeling, and acting. Patients and caregivers in mortal time may be able to move past the moment of diagnosis in ways that allow life's vitality and dignity to be sustained and even enhanced in the shadow of encroaching death. This profound testing requires courage. Art historian James Yood, writing in the preface of *Breast Cancer Journal*, by Hollis Sigler, an artist and breast cancer patient, has captured such courage well in his tribute to her: "This is the particular wonder of Hollis Sigler, to look squarely into the face of mortality and see it as an aperture between promise and despair."[15] Sigler painted in order to capture a kind of preoccupation with one's mortality that often proves the most serious threat to a life of quality in mortal time. Spending too much time contemplating cancer statistics can lead to obsession with death and dying. Patients with a diagnosis of cancer may be unable to live fully in the present because they are understandably preoccupied with the results of the next diagnostic test. The feared possible future of relentless disease dominates and diminishes the present moment. What is needed in these moments? A compassionate, receptive, and reflective posture toward mortality buoys us up in the swells of despair and stops impending death from wiping out life's meaning.

Velma, a 72-year-old woman who had been treated for acute leukemia, had gone through her initial treatment and follow-up care over a period of two years. She had sustained one relapse and following the completion of her second round of chemotherapy was judged to be disease free. However, when the disease returned and she had a third round of chemotherapy, it failed. When her physician sat with her and explained that there were no more good treatment options, Velma began to plan for the remaining days of her life. From her hospital bed she began to call relatives, friends, and loved ones to her bedside. While conscious, alert, and in no pain, she was able to talk openly with her entire family. Knowing that she was going to die, she embraced the opportunity for final conversation with those she loved. Her remarkable courage became a life-sustaining force not only for her family and friends, but also for the entire team on the medical unit where she stayed. She died peacefully, free of pain, in the company of loving caregivers. She died in full awareness of the heartbreak and blessing of mortal time.

Velma's perspective was remarkable. But even genuine receptivity to death cannot substitute for the mundane coping that constitutes most of the day-to-day activity of those living in mortal time. In fact, ordinary activities often bring those who are dying up short, as their purpose is repeatedly called into question. What is the point of taking out the trash when one is dying? Because it piles up, making living uncomfortable and unpleasant. The need to sweep the floor and pay the bills does not go away in mortal time, and such tasks may actually enhance living.

Living in Mortal Time

People in mortal time often move back and forth from everyday coping to thoughts and feelings about the possibility of impending death. Reflective moments do not occur only in religious settings or while gazing out on a beautiful mountain vista. They occur regularly, surprisingly, and not always pleasantly.

One of our patients had a recurrence of colon cancer; it had spread to her liver. She knew that it was not curable. One evening in a heated exchange she commented angrily and sarcastically to her husband, "Well, you won't have to worry about me for very much longer!"

She was aware of intense feelings crashing through as she confronted her "death sentence" in mortal time. Yet she was not able to keep them from surfacing angrily with loved ones. Nor should she have. Anger is a most human response to loss and needs to be heard and held by caregivers in mortal time.

People facing death often comment that distraction or change that takes them away from their ordinary routine helps them to avoid intrusive thoughts about their life-threatening illness. However, one can't remain distracted forever. In the words of Jon Kabat-Zinn, "Wherever you go, there you are."[16] We cannot escape ourselves; we take our thoughts and feelings with us wherever we go. While the most powerful distractions are often the simplest of activities—watching a child at play, taking part in a game of cards, reading a novel, or celebrating a family holiday—those who are dying and their caregivers cannot escape fleeting thoughts and anxieties amidst the everydayness of their lives. A painful paradox of mortal time, in fact, is that mundane events often call to mind and heart what will be lost to the death that is approaching. Living deeply in any situation means facing into what is really happening.

This is as true for those of us living in ordinary time as for those who have entered into mortal time. The latter, however, no longer have the luxury of avoiding or denying the inevitability of death through the illusion of endless time.

Many patients and their caregivers shuttle back and forth, in and out, of acute mortal time over a lengthy period. The initial diagnoses of a life-threatening illness like cancer, followed by a failed treatment, or perhaps a series of failed treatments, are all painful reminders of the march of the disease. However, there are often long periods of remission where life without symptoms is restored. During these periods, people may leave behind the acute subjective experience of mortality and find the illusion of endless time temporarily, albeit partially, restored. Indeed, many types of cancer are like chronic illnesses, to be managed over long periods of time. The experience of mortality becomes definitive only when all treatment options have been exhausted and the disease is free to run its course. Encountering a trauma such as the prospect of fatal illness inevitably shakes and tests what we have taken for granted. Thus, at a time when we most long for stability, all that we have taken for granted is assaulted by the prospect of death. Personal assumptions that have never been challenged are often shattered in mortal time.

Mary Jane had assumed that her bone marrow transplantation would eradicate her breast cancer for good. Her deep faith, strong web of supportive relationships, healthy lifestyle, and "high tech" medical care were all powerful forces contributing to her cure. She was a fighter and badly shaken when the cancer returned. She faced a nagging question that challenged her fundamental belief: "Did I not have enough faith? Did I not believe strongly enough that God could heal me?" She told her caregiver that she had to recast her own story and assumptions about the power of faith to cure, wrestling now with an ancient question: Why me?

The experience of mortal time is profoundly personal. What death means to the dying and their caregivers, and, therefore, how they feel and act in facing it, depends upon the assumptions they bring and how successfully they collaborate in facing what confronts them. Mary Jane's failed treatment shattered an unnamed, implicit assumption: "If I have enough faith, I will be healed."

Sources of Hope

For many patients and caregivers, the ultimate source of hope is in spirituality. Bob Stone, author with Jenny Stone Humphries of the memoir *Where the Buffaloes Roam,* had a very aggressive form of cancer that had spread. He spoke of his situation as follows: "I know I can't be cured of my disease. But I am healed emotionally and spiritually. This healing is every bit as powerful as cure; it's just on a different plane."[17] He drew hope from a spirituality in which physical cure is only one possibility. Bob's view of the world allowed him to interpret and feel death as a process of entering the next world. The hope of Mary, whom you met in our introduction, clearly resided in her religious faith. Her belief and sense of what was happening to her were nearly inconceivable to the young physician-in-training who was treating her, because his source of hope was different—the rational, scientific paradigm where truth is determined by experimental research. Different life experiences create different assumptions and diverse sources of hope.

Nevertheless, There Is Meaning

What can anchor us, when we feel the tug of despair in mortal time? Early in his career, a student came to see the great teacher and philosopher Martin Buber. Failing to read between the lines, Buber did not realize until too late that the young man had come to him on the verge of despair, "not for a chat but for a decision." Upon learning of the subsequent death of his student, Buber asked himself what a human being expects when reaching out to another person in the attempt to ward off despair. His magnificent answer echoes down through the years: "Surely a presence by means of which we are told that, nevertheless, there is meaning."[18] When death's imminent approach undercuts normal, everyday expectations of the future, patients and caregivers alike need reassurance that meaning and hope endure. We discuss a most potent source of that reassurance in Part II—Hope from Conversation.

PART II

Hope from Conversation

There can be no hope which does not constitute itself through
a we and for a we . . . I would be very tempted to say that
all hope is at bottom choral.[1]

— GABRIEL MARCEL[1]

HOPE FOR THE DAY

Mortal time arrives when death's possible approach has
been announced in the form of a life-threatening diagnosis.
There is no turning back. Someone is facing the prospect of
death, and those involved know it. Knowing that some
people defy the medical odds and recover does not alter
the likely outcome for everyone else, and may in fact result
in a type of avoidance that helps no one. How individuals
keep hope alive in the face of imminent mortality, as we
noted in Part I, depends largely upon the personal assumptions they bring from past experience. The other major
contributors to the meaning-making process in mortal time
are caregivers. Professionals in medicine, mental health, and

ministry, along with volunteers, family members, and friends can help someone facing life-threatening illness gather meaning and value from a situation in which many find only despair. They do so by their willingness to be attentive, listen compassionately, and speak openly but tactfully with the one who is facing the possibility of death. They listen carefully and respond thoughtfully.

As we discussed in Part I, the critical underlying challenge for patients and caregivers in mortal time is maintaining a sense of hope. The philosopher Gabriel Marcel captures the relational nature of hope by saying that it is constituted "through a *we* and for a *we*." America's legendary emphasis on individualism too often obscures the truth that living—and dying—inevitably unfold in the company of others, for better and for worse. Nowhere is this awareness more important than in mortal time. Maintaining or losing hope is not an individual feat or failure, but rather something that we do together, in relationships. The great Czechoslovakian writer and statesman Vaclav Havel said, "Hope is definitely not the same thing as optimism. It is not the conviction that something will turn out well, but the certainty that something makes sense, regardless of how it turns out . . . . Hope is a feeling that life and work have meaning."[2] The key phrase here is "regardless of how it turns out." The outcome of serious illness may be death. Making peace and accepting this reality does not eradicate but rather gives birth to another form of hope— hope for meaning even in the midst of this.

Incurable disease can undermine or eliminate the hope that many of us operate on each day, that is, the natural hope of life extending into a distant future. Abrupt removal of that hope is devastating. For those who have entered mortal time, hope can mean the possibility of getting back to the old days, the way things used to be, getting back to normal. But entering a period of chronic, incurable illness eliminates that possibility for many people. Paradoxically, this can give those walking together in mortal time access to new and deeper wellsprings of hope.

Mandy was a long-time breast cancer survivor. She had learned what she said "really mattered" through managing numerous recurrences and treatments over eight years. When asked how she managed her cheerful demeanor and daily motivation, she said, "Of course there are many things that help me, including my friends and my work. It helps a great deal to have something to look forward to, setting goals. I have little goals on most days and long-term goals also. Paddling down the Colorado River had always been a dream, but when I turned it into a goal it really helped me focus positively for a matter of months as we prepared for the trip. Having something to look forward to makes a big difference each and every day."

Mandy's words make it clear that hopeful goals pulled her forward and helped her avoid being trapped by invasive thoughts about dying that could overwhelm her. She figured out that the most significant threat to the quality of her present life was not the prospect of death, but rather intrusive thoughts about what might happen in the future. Setting goals for living helped her avoid this common mortal-time dilemma.

AVOIDING GLOOM

Gloom-and-doom partners are not the best companions in mortal time. However, talking about incurable, life-threatening illness and death is serious business and elicits subtle variations of many different emotions, including fear, anxiety, and anger. It is usually best to begin conversations in mortal time by paying attention to the emotions of the ill person and remaining alert and open to what she or he is feeling before sharing one's own feelings and thoughts. This receptive stance is an invitation to the other to say what's on his or her mind. Talking about dying is hard. Yet, when the prospect of mortality is called sharply into focus, it need not obscure hope.

FALSE HOPE

It is not uncommon in medical settings to hear warnings against giving patients "false hope." False hope is thought to occur when the medical team does not eradicate expectations about cure when cure is statistically unlikely, or when members of the team, especially the doctor, avoid talking directly about the likelihood of death. Professional caregivers share a wise wariness about giving unrealistic expectations to patients and family members, lest they feel uninformed if the medical situation should go bad quickly. Unfortunately, this appropriate concern may result in overly dire predictions, or undue emphasis on worst-case scenarios. Would it be wise to hope to be alive for a daughter's high school graduation in twelve months for a patient who has a projected life span of only six months? In such circumstances, how is a caregiver to respond to a question like, "Do you think I can make it to Susan's graduation?" Would it be more humane to say, "We'll give it our best shot" or "That will be a long shot given your disease status at the moment"? Would "giving it our best shot" be giving false hope?

The late Stephen Jay Gould was diagnosed with mesothelioma in 1982 and told that his cancer had an eight-month median mortality rate after discovery. He crafted a pointed response to the predictors of doom entitled "The Median Isn't the Message."[3] Gould, who lived for twenty more years and died of an illness unrelated to mesothelioma, offers a salutary reminder of the limitations and dangers of statistical predictions about the duration of life: "The problem may be briefly stated: What does 'median mortality of eight months' signify in our vernacular? I suspect that most people, without training in statistics, would read such a statement as 'I will probably be dead in eight months'—the very conclusion that must be avoided, since it isn't so, and since attitude matters so much."

CONVERSATION

The word *conversation* comes from two Latin roots: the prefix *con-*, meaning "with," and the verb *vertere*, meaning "to turn." When two or more people converse, they turn their attention to something together. Conversation creates bridges between professional and family caregivers and people in mortal time. Anatole Broyard has called the powerful moment of conversation where the professional caregiver and the patient experience a connection, the "click of contact."[4] This is the instant when eyes meet and understanding passes between two people in a powerful, compassionate, wordless exchange. In that "click," the patient becomes more than a bed number on rounds, an example of a diagnostic category, or a crisis to be managed; the caregiver becomes more than an objective outsider. Now two human beings have connected face to face. This can indeed be an opening for a "healing conversation," or may remain an unspoken moment of deep human connection. Even a few such moments of deep mutual acknowledgment can make a very big difference to anxious patients.[5]

These moments of acknowledgement are particularly important when the reality of mortal time presses in and why the calling of the professional or family caregiver is such a life giving challenge.

Bill was familiar with the look on Dr. Thomas' face when he entered the exam room with bad news. He knew what might be coming by the look on his physician's face before he said a word. Bill knew that the news was not good, and he deeply appreciated this special moment with his physician, who knew what he had to do in order to tell Bill the truth of his situation. Dr. Thomas would pause for a moment to give him a chance to catch his breath and read the nonverbal cues. The news was not good, but the caring physician acknowledged the gravity of the moment, not so much with what he said but by his manner and presence when entering the exam room where he must tell his patient that the treatment was not working, that the cancer was advancing.

This dramatic encounter between Bill and his physician highlights the importance of nonverbal communication when talking about life-threatening circumstances. It is both **what** is said and **how** it is said that can make a difference. Next we consider the nature of healing conversation and provide general guidelines for the process of talking and listening in mortal time

HEALING CONVERSATION: BASIC ELEMENTS

Everyday conversation can become both more important and more complicated when one of the partners has entered mortal time. The personal assumptions and histories of patients and caregivers set in motion a rhythm of conversation between them that has the power to generate consolation and hope for both. Or they can produce polite civility, collusion in denying the severity of the patient's condition and the caregiver's real response to it, leaving the parties in minimal, uncomfortable contact. Differences in personal assumptions and histories can also result in open conflict and alienation at this worst possible time. We offer the following practical guidelines based on our experience as conversation partners for those who wish to communicate well in mortal time.

Healing conversation has two basic requirements. The more deeply we accept both, the richer the communication that will result. The first is that we grasp our conversation partner's take on things; we "get" what's happening as he or she feels and sees it. **We listen carefully.** Understanding another means seeing a situation from his or her point of view. *Empathy* is one word for such understanding. To empathize is to grasp both the events and the feelings conveyed through another's story, to make a disciplined effort to set aside our thoughts and feelings and walk in the other's shoes for a time. The events are the facts of the conversation, as delivered in words. Feelings signal emotional tone and intensity. Feelings are usually expressed by how words are spoken, including nonverbal signals, and are much more complex than any transcript of words can capture. Empathy, which we discuss in more depth later, requires both attentive listening and appropriate eye contact to fathom the content and feelings of a patient's communication. Caregivers who can turn toward the subject of death in an empathic manner with those who are facing it invite the possibility of hope-creating conversations.

The second requirement of healing conversation is that we put into words our response to what we have heard. We say what we think, feel, believe, desire, question, and so forth in communicating with another. **We respond thoughtfully and honestly.** The letter to the Ephesians in the Christian scriptures puts this requirement in the simple, challenging form of "speaking the truth in love."[6] Note the double obligation here. "Speak the truth" means call things as we really see them; "in love" means with profound respect for our conversation partner. Anyone taking relationships seriously feels the tension inherent in honest, loving speech. Given the inherent anxiety of the mortal time zone, it may be equally important to "hold the truth in love" at certain times. Something may be true, but that doesn't mean that I can hear it from you right at this moment, no matter how tactfully you put it. For example, it may be true for some patients that "chemotherapy is very hard" or that "a particular type of cancer almost always comes back," but saying that to a person newly arrived in mortal time is likely to be misguided honesty, perhaps betraying a caregiver's discomfort more than a patient's need to know something. Speaking the truth in conversation is a process best informed by experience, compassion, and wisdom. Sometimes professional caregivers mistake probabilities based on statistics for truth.

While the requirements of healing conversation are simple—namely, to listen and respond—the communication process itself is a complex matter of mutual interpretation of facts and feelings. The capacities for language and empathy are wired into human beings. But accurate interpretation and skillful use of language are acquired over many years and will surely be tested in the challenging circumstances of mortal time. As we've noted earlier, even experienced professionals with highly developed communication skills can feel awkward and out of place when encountering someone in mortal time.

TALKING IN AND ABOUT MORTAL TIME

Talking *in* mortal time is different than talking *about* mortal time. The subject matter of conversation partners in mortal time may be explicitly or implicitly about dying, or about other things entirely, depending upon patients' and caregivers' dispositions, abilities, openness, and needs at particular moments. The primary requirement is that both partners enter these conversations with awareness of and respect for the gravity of the situation. Given that attitude, the dance of conversation can take on an endless variety of forms and address any and all relevant subjects. A person may wish to discuss the prospect of death openly and often or be able to make only fleeting references to it. Healing conversation can occur when conversation partners in mortal time are able to tolerate the topic of death without fear that they will be overwhelmed or are "giving up." If acknowledging the possibility of death is considered giving up, then we all must give up in the end. We might better consider it "giving over" to our inevitable destiny, which is not giving up at all.

When Natalie learned about her diagnosis of breast cancer, she was also told that surgery was not recommended. The breast cancer had metastasized to her liver, and it would not be useful to operate. She was told that she had a life span of approximately nine months. She underwent three difficult rounds of chemotherapy that made her very sick. Subsequently, she discontinued her chemotherapy treatments. Surprisingly, her tumor seemed to stabilize. When she came to speak with a professional caregiver, she said, "I was supposed to be dead by now . . . . the problem is despair." She went on to describe many life difficulties, the cancer diagnosis and dismal prognosis being just one of a litany of problems. She wrote eloquently about the importance of discussing this:

"I speak of space—the space where I face death, the space where we talk together . . . capturing the moment, counting the breath, attempting to be in the now. Facing death together. Being in that space."

Not everyone approaches mortal time like Natalie, with a poet's keen eye for observing the soul *in extremis.* Doing so provided her with comfort and relief. How is one to respond constructively to such profound self-revelation? Skill is important, but it is compassion expressed through empathy along with tactful honesty that makes *the* difference.

The training and vocation of the professional caregiver allow for openness to talking about death as one way of sustaining hope, but without forcing the issue. A possible conversation opener initiated by a professional caregiver in this spirit is as follows: "Most people who are diagnosed with your illness have some worries about death and dying. We can talk about it whenever you want and leave it alone when you don't." Such a simple invitation is often met with relief since patients and caregivers alike can vacillate between being reluctant to speak of the possibility of death and being unable to speak of anything else. These are hard, necessary healing conversations that require courage and hope. Few people approach talking about mortality with the fortitude of Natalie without a good conversation partner.

CONVERSATION PARTNERS

People coping with the acute experience of mortal time need good health care and appropriate medications as part of the treatment formula. Equally important is tending to the emotional and spiritual needs of vulnerable people in mortal time through supportive companionship. It is a rare patient or caregiver who is not greatly distressed by the diagnosis of a life-threatening illness. The words that are used in these life-changing diagnostic encounters can stay with people for a lifetime, for better or worse. We all have heard examples of health-care practitioners being curt and insensitive. One patient told of her physician's bedside manner. He was trying to be encouraging on the day after her mastectomy by quoting from Shakespeare's *Julius Caesar*: "Cowards die many times before their deaths; the valiant never taste of death but once."[7] Her spirits were low; she was uncomfortable and not in the mood for pep talk from a surgeon quoting the words of a Roman general. Any caregiver will have bad days when caring for patients, but fortunately most are skillful, caring professionals who do their best to provide accurate information in a compassionate, respectful manner.

Family, friends, clergy, and health professionals are ordinarily the primary conversation partners of people in mortal time. Words cannot change the facts of the situation, but they can decisively shape how the situation is experienced and allow for mutual expression of feelings. Knowledgeable professionals are in a position to give accurate information respectfully; family and friends are in a position to listen deeply to the hurt and fear of patients who may be experiencing what can become an overwhelming sense of loss. Healing occurs in mortal time when a caregiver takes in the experience of his or her suffering companion with compassion and acknowledges it honestly, thereby sharing for a moment the burden of mortality. Here, we think of the simple saying "A burden shared is but half a trouble." Having a companion in mortal time, to "just listen and talk" about anything and everything, the light and the heavy, is a healing elixir. We say more about such companionship in Part III.

The basic requirements for conversation that sustains hope are empathy and honesty. Every one of us has the capacity for both, and all of us can deepen those capacities. Mortal time brings the challenge and opportunity to do just that. We turn now to a deeper look at these basic requirements, first to empathy, then to honesty.

EMPATHY

Empathy is a quality and a specific behavior that allows one to enter the world of another. The experience of receiving empathy can put people in touch with their own voices, in touch with themselves.[8] It is a skill to put feelings of compassion into action. Learning to be empathic requires two steps. First, we must accurately grasp **what** the other person is going through and **how** they are feeling about it. Then, we must convey our understanding to them in some way, let them know that we "get it." Sometimes this can be done by a simple reflection back to the other of what we have heard in the simplest language possible. Sometimes words are unnecessary and a compassionate nod of the head or touch of the hand is sufficient.

Empathy can be powerful medicine for several reasons. First, those fortunate enough to have good listeners for caregivers can hear themselves talk about their situations and perhaps gain new insight. By listening with empathy, caregivers can clarify their own assumptions and interpretations of the situation, which is always a valuable outcome, and never more so than in mortal time. This insight and clarification can lead to problem-solving action, as complicated as coming to some resolution about the existential question "Why me?" or as practical as deciding on a scarf rather than a wig for a head covering. Putting experiences into words can open up new understanding and possibilities for people walking together in mortal time. Extending empathy in this manner, allowing the speaker to confide without interruption or giving back information or an opinion on his or her situation is not easy. The listener may have a natural tendency to attempt to relieve the suffering of another by responding quickly, by shutting off feelings of sadness or distress. The person who says "I am scared" may immediately get a response that directs the conversation away from these feelings, like, "Be strong; you can get through this." Such a response, while not inappropriate when spoken at the right moment, can short-circuit the empathic connection before it is set. Further, naming the source of anxiety and fear often encountered in mortal time can relieve suffering. As we noted earlier, entry into mortal time can be abrupt and frightening. Naming fear is the first step toward mastery of it. With mastery can come relief, at least temporarily. Being in the company of a listener who is extending empathy is strong medicine. Yet, it is not easy to find deep empathy for something one has never before experienced, as a cancer center volunteer wisely noted on her way to becoming "properly empathetic."

BECOMING PROPERLY EMPATHETIC

During her long journey as a volunteer caregiver and courageous cancer survivor, Nina Ann Stokes put it this way: "I
was never really properly empathetic until I experienced the
side effects of chemotherapy."[9] These words by a wise
woman illustrate a common human dilemma. We cannot
directly experience the life of another, but we can do so
indirectly through the quality of our empathy. Even after
eight years of treatment for breast cancer that had recurred
several times, as well as very active volunteer work with
many patients, Nina Ann was learning what it was like to
have numbness in her hands and feet, a hallmark side effect
of some chemotherapy drugs. She was deepening her
already considerable empathy by self-reflection and self-
examination.

Listening carefully and respectfully allows one person
to understand the experience of the other. The limits of our
empathy are determined in part by our ability to allow
differences to register. The caregiving companion with no
experience of incurable illness may be lost when encountering a friend whose father has just died. How is one to
empathize with an unknown experience? Can we truly
understand someone when we haven't been through what
they are facing? Nancy, a volunteer in our cancer patient

support program and a "veteran" patient of two different cancers, says that without going through a cancer diagnosis, it is impossible to really understand what it is like. She emphatically says, "You just cannot understand unless you have been there." We look at this differently. No one fully comprehends what another is going through, not even survivors who have been diagnosed with the same life-threatening illness, although they may have insights that non-patients cannot grasp. Listening deeply to a loved one and responding with empathy brings us as close as we can get to forms of suffering that we have not experienced directly ourselves. Vicarious experience is limited, but real.

Experience with an illness and treatment-related side effects may help in deepening empathic capacity. However, even if two people have the same diagnosis and treatment, both will go through a unique situation because of differences in their personal assumptions. The meaning of a cancer diagnosis will be interpreted by each person uniquely, and those meanings differ. An example of misguided empathic connecting is the patient who has had a bad experience with chemotherapy and assumes that it will be that way for everyone. Some people manage chemotherapy with virtually no side effects and miss no work, while others are nearly incapacitated by a similar course of treatment. This probably is related to differing metabolic rates and other biological responses to chemotherapy drugs that vary among individuals, as well as personal history and the quality of available supportive relationships. While one's own experience is a good teacher, it does not hold the only key to understanding.

RECEIVING EMPATHY

Expressions of empathy may not be received as intended. One of us once consulted with a wise, caring physician as he met with a couple to discuss treatment planning. The chemotherapy approach so far had not been working, and the patient's disease was progressing; it was a turning point in treatment, where neither cure nor containment was possible. The very aggressive cancer was advancing in spite of all best efforts. In gentle and clear fashion, the physician laid out his plan: there would be no more chemotherapy recommended, as it would only make the patient sick and would not stop the disease. The patient sat stunned, with his wife sitting next to him and crying quietly as she began to grasp the gravity of their situation. Cure was not possible. We sat for nearly fifteen minutes with this couple while the oncologist continued explaining his reasoning for the recommendation. A check later in the day to see how the patient was doing revealed that he had been discharged early. Within the next week, at the patient's follow-up appointment, this surprising exchange took place: "That was a very difficult conversation we had in the hospital. How are you doing with all that?" The patient's answer was astonishing: "He told me and just left." The patient's experience of this exchange was that the physician gave him information and then abruptly left. In reality, the physician had spent a significant amount of time with the couple even though it was a very busy day of rounds in the hospital. But in such situations, the "facts" of the matter do not matter. What one of us had observed contradicted what the patient experienced. He felt abandoned. This story underscores the complexity of interchanges in mortal time and the challenge to caregivers to listen carefully and communicate what they hear tactfully to the patient. What could the physician have done differently? Perhaps he could have stopped talking to wait, even if just for a moment, for the patient or spouse to respond. Silent presence or just waiting is very difficult for most caregivers, both professional and nonprofessional. Most people act quickly to fill silent space out of their own discomfort. It is the rare caregiver who can stifle the urge to respond quickly, to make things better, to take away the pain, an impossible task. But even if he had paused, the patient may still have felt abandoned. There are limits to what a person can do in these moments of contact.

Even when one does listen carefully and respond compassionately, the patient may not receive it that way. In all human relationships, and especially those unfolding in mortal time, it is good to remember sociologist W. I. Thomas's maxim about the human condition: "A situation which is perceived as real will be real in its effects."[10] In this case the patient perceived that his physician had given him bad news and left abruptly, and yet another observer, the consultant, saw a different reality. Both perceptions had real effects. This underscores the importance of the second basic requirement for conversation in mortal time after empathy: honesty.

HONESTY: WHAT CAN I SAY?

"I don't know what to say. I don't know what I should say. And, he doesn't know what to say to me." These poignant words came from David, a father unable to speak to his son in the face of the boy's incurable illness. They illustrate one very important question for anyone accompanying someone through the diagnosis and treatment of a life-threatening illness: What can I say? Most people have little practice at this, and even experienced professionals are often at a loss for words. Arrival in mortal time often renders words hollow. Consequently, we feel inadequate, don't know what to say, or when to say it, and may avoid the topic of what's happening to our friend or loved one altogether because we simply can't find good words. Even if we find the right words, can we then make them words well spoken?

As we've noted, the second requirement of conversation is responding thoughtfully and truthfully. Many caregivers get stuck on "the right thing to say." They worry that they won't have the right words and often look to experts to supply them. While it is true that people who have companioned others in mortal time extensively may have suggestions, every person with the ability to empathize can find their own words to meet the situation. Sometimes there is no need for words: an attentive presence and a caring silence are all that is required. For the professional medical caregiver, telling the truth is complicated even more by the ambiguity of medical information and the reality that fact and truth may not be exactly the same. While the facts of the situation may indicate a limited life span due to advanced disease, the truth of the matter for an individual may unfold quite differently. In these circumstances, professional honesty means understanding and communicating at the proper time both the best and the worst that can happen.

THE RIGHT WORDS

Words can take strange twists in mortal time, and not only for caregivers. A patient spoke poignantly of the challenge in communicating about his fatal diagnosis with his spouse and adult sons:

> *"I knew she didn't know that there really was no cure, no magic bullet, unless the man upstairs decides to send a miracle. But I didn't know how to tell her. She only understood today when we talked to the doctor again. . . . But my son doesn't know. He is busy with his school, which has been very good to him, letting him postpone a test when I was so sick. I think I should tell him. I know this will be hard for him; I do not want to hurt him. . . . I need to tell my son about this; it needs to come from me."*

These are the words of a loving husband and father trying to shield his wife and son from the pain and suffering caused by the prospect of his dying. In this situation, he is searching for the right time and the right words to speak the truth to his wife and son about his harsh and sudden entry into mortal time and impending death at age 58. He wants a real conversation with his loved ones and knows that it will be painful on all sides. He wants to make emotional contact by talking about his situation, and yet as a good father and husband wants to protect his loved ones. He knew that his honesty would lead to suffering, yet his courage moved him toward acknowledgment of his sudden entry into what would likely be a short life in mortal time.

ACKNOWLEDGING FEAR

Anxiety and uncertainty are conversation blockers, and never more so than in mortal time. If we assume that a person coping with a life-threatening diagnosis is fearful and does not want to talk about his or her illness, we could either avoid the topic altogether or jump right in anyway. The former could result in uncomfortable efforts to ignore the proverbial elephant in the room; the latter can give rise to heavy-handed blunders like, "How do you feel about dying?" This question was asked by a coworker of a person newly diagnosed with early-stage prostate cancer, hardly a candidate for dying. In a misguided effort to say something, the coworker stuck his foot deeply into his mouth. Fortunately, the patient was not hurt but rather dumfounded by the insensitivity of this inquiry. In fact, it is rare for all but the closest relatives and health-care team members to be in conversation with a patient who is literally on his or her "death bed." Most caregivers meet people who are living in a less acute experience of mortal time, where death is not imminent. It is difficult if not impossible to predict the hour, day, week, month, or even year of one's death in all but the most grave of circumstances.[11]

Caregivers may see deep sadness and anxiety in their loved ones and reflexively want to soothe them. Paradoxically, some attempts to comfort may compound suffering by distancing companions in mortal time from the issues at hand. For example, a common tendency of well-meaning family members is to say, "Let's not talk that way; don't give up now" in response to a person who says with a fearful sad tone, "This cancer is going to get me in the end." Family caregivers may be extremely anxious, sad, or depressed themselves and unable to tolerate conversation that directly acknowledges the prospect of loss. Such situations often call for a particular and demanding kind of communication at a time when the conversation partner feels inadequate and even paralyzed. Both empathy and information may need to be communicated—empathy for what the person is feeling and information to correct misconceptions. Cancer may well *not* "get you" in the end. Nevertheless, at this point in the conversation it is important to acknowledge the fear by responding with empathy first and encouragement later as appropriate. For example, a caregiver might respond with an empathic statement ("You sound sad and really worried about what's happening") and encouragement ("We are in this together; let's just see what we can do"). Caregivers who aren't experienced in the art of listening carefully and responding thoughtfully may be quick to encourage and not to empathize, missing the deep interpersonal connection that can develop from such acknowledgement.

EVERYDAY CONVERSATION WITH FRIENDS

One sensitive survivor of initial diagnosis as well as recurrent episodes of cancer speaks of how important conversation with an extended circle of friends can be. He suggests that people continue to behave as normally as possible, include the cancer patient survivor in gatherings, and continue "slap-on-the-back" greetings. It is of course important to be mindful of a person's health situation but equally important not to dwell on it. This is a delicate, shifting series of judgment calls differing from one person to another, and from moment to moment with the same person. Some people welcome the opportunity for head-on, frank talk about their condition, while others dismiss inquiries with simple responses like, "I'm hangin' in there." Momentous as it is, the diagnosis and treatment of a life-threatening illness is only one subplot in a much larger life. Other topics of conversation are important as well. Knowing what is timely for mortal-time conversations requires a kind of disciplined spontaneity. Mistakes will be made, and there is no shame in that.

Sometimes, though, those in need of empathy are met with platitudes, or are simply ignored entirely. All too often well-meaning friends and loved ones may be oblivious to the suffering around them or unprepared to respond to it. Even a silent presence can offer comfort, as Anton Chekhov wisely illustrated in the short story "Misery—To Whom Shall I Tell My Grief?"[12] In the story, Iona, a carriage driver, repeatedly tries to tell the story of his son's death to several of his passengers, who either ignore him completely or chastise him. As the story concludes, Iona is feeding his faithful horse at the end of the long cold night. The horse is attentive and hears the story of Iona's son's death. "The little mare munches, listens, and breathes on her master's hands. Iona is carried away and tells her all about it." His horse extends listening to her master in a way that none of Iona's human companions that night would.

All Iona needed was to give words to his grief in the presence of listening.

PLATITUDES: LET'S HOPE FOR THE BEST AND PREPARE FOR THE WORST

The natural tendency for many people—*especially* health-care professionals, who are trying to be helpful to patients in difficult circumstances—is to respond with such platitudes as "Hang in there" or "Just take one day at a time." A specific platitude may become habitual for a health-care professional or someone who regularly comes in contact with the frightened or bereaved. A once-in-a-lifetime event for the patient or family caregiver may be a daily experience for the professional using routine phrases to comfort, and certain platitudes may take on a ritualized quality. "Let's hope for the best and prepare for the worst" can become a constantly repeated line in the daily practice of cancer physicians, who commonly see patients with very difficult medical circumstances. It could be recited many times in one day by the medical practitioner, and yet it might be the first time a patient or family has heard it. Nonetheless, the words may be comforting for both the caregiver and the patient or family member. The statement is usually very well received by most patients. Sometimes those with a spiritual sensibility add "and pray for a miracle."

A caregiver who lovingly accompanied his wife through an extremely difficult and painful breast cancer treatment said, "A bad platitude is better than running away." His own faithful companionship with his spouse in mortal time allowed him to present a basic ground rule for all who dwell in mortal time: show up and be present; make the effort to reach out, even when uncomfortable. As this caregiver learned, being there is the key. Platitudes may sound hollow and shallow, or inspirational and uplifting, depending on the manner in which they are offered and the assumptions of those receiving them. Some common phrases used to comfort are:

> *There are no cancers that someone hasn't beaten.*
> *Cancer is no match for you.*
> *Tomorrow will be a better day.*
> *Miracles do happen.*
> *You can get through anything.*
> *This too shall pass.*
> *God has a plan for you.*
> *God does not give you more than you can take.*
> *Let's hope for the best, prepare for the worst, and pray for a miracle.*
> *Things happen for a reason.*

Live one day at a time.
This is a marathon, not a sprint.
Time will tell.

This small sample of platitudes is heard regularly by those in mortal time. They may be comforting and useful to the person who simply does not know what to say. All too often, however, the effect of using platitudes to avoid the awkwardness of being with someone who is anxious and suffering is to put distance between the conversation partners. While a patient may come to the conclusion that such platitudes as "Everything happens for a reason" can be comforting, this may not be his or her immediate response. One patient told us that she was deeply offended and angered when, during the diagnostic interview, her oncologist offered that, "Your cancer is a gift to you; it will help you set priorities, and it will change your life." Again, while this may be true, and this patient actually decided after much reflection that it was, during the early diagnostic period it was an insult. "How dare you tell me that a diagnosis of cancer is a gift in the midst of anxiety and worry," she felt like telling her oncologist. Only patients themselves can conclude that cancer is a gift: that perspective cannot be shoehorned. Just as drug dosages require adjustments based on patient characteristics like weight, so too the type of conversation cannot be limited to a formula where all patients hear the same words. The timing and "dosing" of language in mortal time is an art.

Other platitudes are sobering and jarring; they can frighten and do harm, depending on who is speaking, how the phrases are said, and when and where they are spoken. Some examples are:

> *If you have to have a cancer, this is a good one to have.*
> *Everybody has to go sometime, we are all going to die.*
> *If I were you, I would be taking all of my vacation time.*
> *You can't take it with you.*
> *You could get hit by a bus at any time.*
> *I have been working here a long time and have learned how quickly things can change.*
> *Let me put it this way: you had better get your affairs in order.*
> *There is no hurry to have surgery; that cancer has probably been developing in your breast for years.*
> *Hard times build character.*
> *Not everybody dies of that, you know.*

YOU FIRST!

Platitudes can be used for better or worse, and sometimes patients repeat well-worn phrases to themselves, such as "Just hang in there." It is not uncommon for people to refer to their own mortality in the following manner: "Well, you can't live forever." This cavalier statement made in casual conversation among the healthy is generally harmless. But when a physician casts a remark like this at a person facing life-threatening illness, it can be harmful. A caregiver tells the story of learning of her husband's dire prognosis during his stay in the intensive care unit. After a conversation in which the physician laid out the dismal prospects for her husband, he commented in what seemed to her all too casually, "We all have to go sometime," to which she replied, "You first!" The sensitive, experienced caregiver companion, whether professional or family member, knows when to offer a useful platitude and when to remain silent, yet deeply present.

THE HUMANE USE OF WORDS: EFFECTIVE PHRASES IN MORTAL TIME

The ethical principles guiding the humane use of words are first "do no harm" and then "try to do good." There are many words and phrases that caregivers may use in the spirit of these principles; such words can be used to extend kindness and comfort. The following phases used alone as simple statements of connection or together with other statements in conversation can be used to comfort:

> *I am with you in this . . .*
> *This is very difficult territory . . .*
> *We can get through this . . .*
> *You can count on me . . .*
> *I am sorry you are going through this . . .*
> *Can you tell me how you are holding up?*
> *How can I be useful?*

Such phrases, stated with genuineness and empathy, invite further conversation rather than closing off meaningful dialogue. A person who can listen carefully and respond thoughtfully with simple, direct statements like these has the power to help lower the emotional distress encountered in mortal time.

CONSIDERATION AND DISCIPLINED SPONTANEITY

Most people are not comfortable talking with friends and relatives about life-threatening illness or the possibility of dying, and often turn to professionals or self-help books for advice. The father whose statement we quoted—"I don't know what to say. I don't know what I should say. And, he doesn't know what to say to me."—illustrated the initial awkwardness that most people experience in the mortal time zone. Most people can discover the words, if they can find the courage and manage their anxiety, for conversation in mortal time. As we discussed earlier, the basic ground rules for respectful communication do not change in mortal time even though the topics of conversation may be much more difficult to face. In the everyday give-and-take of conversation, spontaneity is one life-giving element, a source of much joy for human beings. However, spontaneous comments without some disciplined consideration of the psychological and spiritual state of those facing the possibility of death can cause unintended pain. It is not uncommon for a well-meaning friend or relative to respond without consideration to a person facing life-threatening illness. The listener tries to reach out but does so in a spontaneous and harmful way. The following story illustrates **spontaneity without consideration.**

> *Sheila's new diagnosis of breast cancer had come as a shock to her. However, after her initial surgical treatment she was adjusting reasonably well even with the prospect of chemotherapy ahead*

of her. She recounted that she had been describing her scheduled
treatment and how she was doing so far to a friend. The friend
proceeded to blurt out: "Well my aunt had breast cancer and
chemotherapy too. The chemotherapy was unbelievably difficult.
It almost killed her. She did live several years after that and then
her cancer came back. It always comes back."

Sheila was stunned and frightened by her friend's comments, an example of a spontaneous and thoughtless statement. A volunteer in our cancer center tells of overhearing the following comment spoken by a caregiver of one patient to another patient in the waiting area: "Oh, my mother had that and she was gone in three weeks." It is not difficult to imagine how such words might affect a person just beginning chemotherapy. This unsolicited input is clearly unwarranted and surely unwanted. It is an excellent example of "foot in mouth" syndrome that can occur when someone does not know what to say and blurts out whatever comes to mind.

With some embarrassment and obvious remorse, a very thoughtful and spontaneous practitioner tells the following story. One of his patients had undergone more than one course of radiation therapy. Unfortunately, her tumors returned on several occasions. During an office visit, her physician, in a moment of spontaneous and light exchange commented, "You are just a little tumor-making machine, aren't you?" Several months later, when the patient screwed up her courage and told him how that comment had hurt and scared her, he was embarrassed and self-critical. He had intended the comment to be humorous and upon reflection was surprised at his own tactless question to her, saying, "How could I have said that?" We all have tactless moments; however, not all caregivers are as mature and open as this practitioner, who had built a relationship of trust that eventually led to another conversation where the comment was discussed, the patient could express her feelings, and he could offer his apology. An apology always helps, no matter how embarrassing it might be to bring up the thoughtless comment.

CENSORED CONVERSATION
vs. ACTIVE LISTENING

On the other end of the continuum of spontaneous interchange is the person who censors all responses containing potentially disturbing information. This results in hesitant, polite, and distant comments devoid of life-giving energy like, "I am sure everything will work out all right."

Compassionate conversation requires spontaneity, consideration, and disciplined understanding of the person's situation. This skill demands active, careful listening first before responding with words. Of course, the act of being present and attentive is a very powerful and healing response in and of itself. Companions in mortal time must do their best to listen with compassion and speak the truth in love.

The best intentions to remain calm and open in the presence of a suffering loved one can dissolve in tears or give way to mute anxiety when the caregiver is confronted with the stark possibility of a loved one dying. When someone we care about says, "There is no cure now; the cancer is moving. Is there any hope?" any caregiver will be challenged to find a spontaneous yet disciplined and helpful response. Sometimes, simply saying, "I am so sorry. . . ." is enough.

Professional caregivers may learn how to be disciplined and helpful due to the many opportunities they have to respond to patients with life-threatening illness. Their challenge will be to remain spontaneous. Family caregivers may be spontaneous yet have little experience, undisciplined in the nuances of healing conversation

HOW MUCH TIME DO I HAVE?

One of the more difficult conversations involves the person for whom cure is no longer possible. "How much time do I have, doctor?" is a question that most people with a diagnosis of any life-threatening illness consider asking.[13] Some ask it directly. This is no time for hollow platitudes, and it is important for professional caregivers to have some general philosophy on how to answer this question. It is important for people who ask the question to know whether or not they want what they are asking for. One of our physician colleagues replies this way: "Ultimately, only God can answer that question; I can't be absolutely sure as a doctor. But given your type of cancer, and your current status, if you were to ask me how long, I would answer a matter of weeks or months." One physician suggests that the following one-liner of a senior physician is very effective in this situation: "We will see where we are and we'll go from there." This masterful use of words leaves open possibility; the source of its comfort may be its ambiguity. Of course some patients may need more specificity, which is where the art of medicine is so very crucial. Words have the power to comfort and energize or frighten and demoralize. It is very important that the health-care team recognize this and use both kindness and skill in their day-to-day encounters. It is important for professional caregivers to realize that people generally seek and need accurate information about their prospects even when they are not good.[14]

APPRECIATING EVERYDAY CHATTER

People facing incurable illness may need and want a different type of conversation than the usual everyday chatter, since conversation can lose its meaning in mortal time without some acknowledgment of the gravity of the situation. However, all human beings also need the lightness of humor and the peacefulness of quiet contemplation without fear. Conversation can be both "heavy" and "light" when death is on the near horizon. All human beings walk the fine line between heaviness and lightness, between everyday banter and serious discussion; patients and caregivers in mortal time do so in a particularly demanding way. In our experience, most people who lose their emotional balance in mortal time fall on the side of lightness, that is, not fully appreciating that each day may be one's last. Yet, there is no room for harsh judgments on what is best in mortal time. There are times when the immediate reality of a situation is better avoided. As a Peanuts character once proclaimed in articulating the philosophy of "runism": "There is no problem so big it cannot be run away from." There are moments when it is best to run from the painful reality of mortal time, to retreat to the comfort of distraction, perhaps even utilize forms of functional denial.

DENIAL?

It is not uncommon in cancer care to hear, "The patient is in denial." This judgment misses the point that each of us attends selectively to the environment around us. Denial is the psychological process whereby people protect themselves from threatening information by blocking it out of immediate awareness. As such, it is only a more intense form of the selective attention of everyday life. The denial of death is so normal in Western culture that it is often a serious obstacle to real conversation in mortal time. However, it behooves everyone to walk carefully on this territory, never attempting to cram the "reality of the situation" down the throats of people in mortal time. Professional and nonprofessional caregivers often get caught in the expectation that patients should acknowledge and discuss their impending death openly, that they should have "the talk" with their caregivers, that they should "really face" their situation.

Angela had developed pain and shortness of breath as primary symptoms before entering the hospital for a complete diagnostic workup. It was discovered that she had a rare form of sarcoma that had actually grown into the heart muscle, placing her in imminent danger. Furthermore, the prospects of the tumor being responsive to chemotherapy were poor. Her young physician felt that she was in denial, especially when she talked about the distant future with her daughter, who was then in kindergarten. A professional caregiver was asked to speak with her about her denial. In talking with the patient and seeing her somber mood and tears, it was clear that she understood the gravity of the situation. She was petrified by the possibility of leaving her young daughter to fend for herself in the world. However, she was not prepared to discuss her life prospects immediately. She did not want to have "the talk" with the medical team at that point, in that place. Her private nature made her uncomfortable with the regular team rounds, which included up to seven different people standing around her bed early in the morning. However, in a one-to-one conversation it was clear that she understood the seriousness of her situation and the likely outcome.

Professionals can undervalue the importance and use-fulness of avoidance and denial. Some forms of reality, death being one, cannot be integrated quickly. Heartrending situations such as being a single parent unable to protect her child, helpless in the face of relent-less disease, simply cannot be faced easily or quickly without devastating psychological side effects, including the despair we spoke of in Part I. Many family members facing the diagnosis of an illness that can't be cured are understandably at a loss for what to say or do. On the one hand, they desperately cling to hope for a cure and want to be hopeful for the patient. On the other hand, they may instinctively feel a need to talk at deeper levels, to talk about things that matter, to take final chances to commu-nicate with precious loved ones whose lives may be ending. The need to talk about dying and death may be trumped by the social taboo against talking plainly in the face of death as well as by fears of the patient and family members about what to say.

There are many ways to acknowledge death's arrival and many ways in which people protect themselves from the anxiety that accompanies awareness that life is threatened with ending. In Angela's story, the physician felt that she did not truly understand the nature of her situation and that a rational discussion of her impending death was important so that she could tend to last things. He was acting with consideration by calling in the consulting psychologist and had the tact not to push her into "getting her affairs in order" immediately. Yet he felt a responsibility to help her see that her cancer was not curable and could prove fatal soon. Since it had already grown into her heart, it was immediately life threatening in ways that most other cancers are not. The stakes were high and made even more difficult by the fact that the patient was a single mother of a six-year-old daughter who would need to be cared for. Such considerations on the threshold of mortality are gut-wrenching for all involved.

HEALTHY CONVERSATION
ABOUT DYING

There are countless variations of the type of conversation that may emerge in mortal time. The following story illustrates a common one: acknowledging and appreciating a good life together as it ends.

Alice is the older of two children in a loving family. She faced her father's diagnosis and likely fatal prognosis with courage and hope. However, when the disease progressed and left her normally vibrant father bedridden, the inevitable movement of his cancer became painfully evident. Alice longed for a different type of conversation with her father. She wanted to talk with him about his situation and yet he didn't seem to want to talk about death. Perhaps he wanted to protect his daughter and family from what he knew was inevitable. With conviction and courage, Alice raised the issue, asking him to talk to her about their life together. This brave and loving step forward opened the door for deep and intimate conversation between a caring daughter and her loving father in the days before his death. Alice was able to speak deeply and lovingly about their life together, to reminisce about the many years of good times in several conversations at his bedside, and importantly to say her painful and yet life-giving good-bye to her father.

This story shows us what might be gained in an effort to talk about "final things." Such moments offer deep consolation to both parties and treasured, steadying memories for the ones who go on living. In this case Alice courageously and gently spoke with her father about her deep sadness that soon he would no longer be with her. This "death talk" was really a "life talk," a conversation about how much he meant to her and how much she would miss him in the future. Who would she call now about car problems? She had the opportunity, in the midst of tears and laughter, to tell him all that he had meant to her over the years, and to assure him that he would be in her heart forever.

Two important points about these conversations should be underscored. First, not all such attempts end with acceptance and peace. Some people may never want to face the prospect of their own death directly in conversation. They may choose to talk about it in metaphors, speaking of "endings," "moving on," and the like, or not addressing it at all, holding on instead to a stubborn insistence on a miracle. It is the sensitive caregiver who knows how to proceed with such delicate matters, when to push forward and when to remain silent, when to speak the truth in love or hold it in peace. Second, such encounters may happen in less dramatic fashion over a period of weeks, months, or even years.

PRACTICAL CONVERSATION

Direct end-of-life conversation sometimes happens because of practical considerations; for example, the medical team needs to know what patients' wishes are should they be incapacitated.[14] Would they want "everything done" or prefer not to be subjected to the many machines that can prolong life? Because intense emotions are involved here, sometimes what is clear to the medical team is not clear to the family, resulting in prolonged, futile treatment that can actually increase patient and family suffering at the end of life. The entire period between the initial shock of diagnosis to end-of-life conversations involves living in the state of mortal time wherein the awareness of one's finitude becomes more prominent. Walking with loved ones on this terrain can be deeply gratifying and profoundly challenging. One of the demands facing professional caregivers is not to settle for a purely instrumentalist view of an end-of-life conversation, i.e., "Let's get this out of the way," like any ordinary medical procedure. The sensitive task of negotiating orders about resuscitation early in a hospitalization often falls to the least experienced medical providers. This can make for very difficult conversations with distressed patients, uneasy caregivers, and anxious young professionals all struggling on unfamiliar and anxious ground. Such conversations bring all participants—patients and caregivers alike--face to face with their own mortality. How these conversations in mortal time affect caregivers is our subject in Part III.

PART III

GUIDANCE FOR CAREGIVERS

*To everything there is a season and a time to every purpose
under heaven.*[1]
— ECCLESIASTES 3:1

BEING A COMPANION IN MORTAL TIME

There are many different types of companions available to
people cast into mortal time. First and foremost are family
members—a spouse or other partner, parents, siblings,
children, extended family, and friends. Professional caregivers in hospitals and hospices include nurses, physicians,
physician assistants, clergy/chaplains, recreation therapists,
pharmacists, nutritionists, and physical and occupational
therapists. Volunteers from organizations such as hospice
can also be valuable companions. These caregiver companions often become like family during the diagnosis and
treatment of life-threatening illness. Professionals who
regularly work with people in mortal time are in a position

to be "expert companions," special guides who have been there before and know the territory.[2] Friends from work and community may take on important tasks and supportive roles in mortal time. The fundamental task for anyone who would accompany a person in mortal time is becoming a companion.

The word *companion* is derived from the Latin *com,* meaning "together" plus *panis,* meaning "bread." Sharing a meal, or coming together to share bread, is a perfect metaphor for companionship, and bringing a meal to someone remains a simple but profound way of offering companionship in hard times. A companion is one who accompanies another—a comrade, a friend, a conversation partner. Joining with another in companionship is the most powerful antidote to the despair that can accompany profound loss. Perhaps the most basic way that human beings become companions is through conversation. Hope arises from and strengthens a "we."

KIND COMPANIONS

Melissa was hospitalized for many days for treatment of acute leukemia. Growing weary and discouraged, she was physically and emotionally exhausted and had begun ruminating about how bad things were for her. She was stuck in a rut and knew it.

One day a maintenance man told her, "When I get down, I try to think of all the things I am grateful for, and it helps me feel better." She heard this wise advice and began her own form of self-talk, literally changing her thinking by adopting this simple technique of cultivating gratefulness.

Many different people can play an important role in mortal time by offering companionship through small gestures of kindness and compassion. For example, the receptionist in a medical office is often the first person to meet the patient when he or she enters. There are gifted receptionists who have a friendly greeting and smile for all. This sets a tone of warm companionship in a treatment setting. Likewise, housekeeping staff and maintenance staff may have daily contact with hospitalized patients. With a cheerful, gentle demeanor, they make a great deal of difference in the simple exchanges of the day. As Melissa learned, some comments from non-treatment staff can sound a lot like a psychologist's intervention. The many brief conversations that occur around tasks that patients must complete, whether they are hospitalized, coming in for outpatient treatment, or receiving care at home or in hospice, are all potential tiny moments of compassionate companionship.

Ray volunteers every Wednesday morning in an outpatient cancer center where he hosts a hospitality room replete with windows, relaxing music, snacks, and fellowship. He interacts with many patients and family members as they wait for treatment or test results. He listens attentively, remembers details of patient and family lives, and delivers snacks to patients in treatment areas to help with the nausea that can develop. A cancer survivor himself, he often says, "I get so much more than I give. It is my privilege to volunteer."

Being a good companion often means altering your schedule. Dan, an attorney, told us that he was not taking on any new responsibilities or clients in the near future so that he would be available for his wife's anticipated medical appointments and procedures. Her symptoms, including nagging shortness of breath, had become particularly acute over the past three weeks. She had not been able to work or venture too far outside the house, prompting him to increase his availability while managing a busy professional life by necessity as the primary wage earner. He was adjusting as required in order to be a vigilant, faithful companion at a critical moment on this difficult journey where the presence of ever-increasing symptoms seemed to foretell an acceleration of disease progress within mortal time. A particularly difficult psychological task for Dan was to remain present and attentive when the task switched from addressing the episodic acute symptoms of a curable illness to managing the chronic symptoms of an incurable illness. Dan was contending with uncertainty in a way that profoundly affected his every scheduled move. At the same time that he was working mightily to be there for his partner, the feared future was beginning to dawn on him: "I can't help it. . . . I wonder what it might be like to be a widower someday."

Companionship can be made more difficult by complex family circumstances. For example, in a blended family where an ex-spouse is dealing with a life-threatening illness and is geographically separated from children as well as a former spouse, many challenges arise. Communication between the one who is facing mortality and a former spouse can be strained by the prospect of reopening old wounds. This can also be a time of profound healing and forgiveness, and important resolutions that can set free the spirits of the dying and their caregivers for new life after death.

One of us experienced the profoundly moving and healing experience of a last and reconciling conversation with a former spouse, facilitated by our daughter, who had been her mother's faithful caregiver during her terminal illness. She initiated and mediated this final conversation between her parents, holding the phone to her Mom's ear as it unfolded. All three participants felt old burdens lighten. Such are the searing, saving graces of mortal time.

THE COSTS AND RISKS OF COMPANIONSHIP

Being with someone who has entered mortal time produces a dual challenge for caregivers. The first is being compassionately present for the person managing his or her illness. This can be as basic as sitting quietly in a hospital room while waiting for the news following tests, or a more active conversational presence where people talk about the day's events, the meaning of illness, or the patient's possible death. Compassionate presence puts one at risk for absorbing intense suffering. To be open to the suffering of another is to risk personal distress while at the same time bringing grace into the world. This kindness is a form of love in action.

A second challenge is managing the anxiety created when caregivers confront the fact that they too are living in mortal time. Repeated exposure to the thought and experience of mortality is distressing. Social scientists have given this a name: "death anxiety." Such encounters often raise the ultimate questions we raised in Part I: Where did I come from? What is my purpose? What is my destiny? Such questions are not easily answered and may disturb as well as comfort. This is an inherent risk of caring for others in mortal time.

The effects on relationships of encountering suffering in mortal time are cumulative. Faithful companionship in illness can take its toll on any relationship; it will certainly do so when someone is facing his or her own mortality and looming death. The caregiver can literally be worn out by the demands of compassion in the midst of deep suffering. As we noted in Part I, human beings can absorb only so much suffering and anxiety. "Compassion fatigue" is a condition where too much suffering becomes overwhelming. Knowing one's limits as well as knowing how to step back and recharge emotional batteries is an important spiritual discipline for those moving in such trying times. Support and self-care are crucial for those who would be faithful companions in mortal time. At a minimum, good self care includes sufficient food, rest, exercise, and some maintaining of familiar life-giving routines.

THE NINE PERSONAL VIRTUES MOST NEEDED IN MORTAL TIME

It does not take an advanced degree to be a helpful companion in mortal time. It does call for the exercise and often the development of specific qualities that most people have: genuineness, presence, sensitivity, courage, acceptance, respect, compassion, a sense of humor, and awareness of one's own limitations.[3] We use the term "virtue" for these personal qualities, because they are neither techniques nor gimmicks but rather qualities of character that arise from life experience. We all bring virtues to mortal time and may, if we embrace its challenges, deepen old virtues and nurture new ones during these privileged moments.

1. *Genuineness*

Genuineness used here refers to the quality of being oneself. Being in the presence of someone in mortal time may create self-consciousness and embarrassment. There may be moments of silence as well as awkward conversation, especially if the conversation partners are only acquaintances. However, feeling uncomfortable does not negate the possibility of being genuine—in fact, it may facilitate deeper forms of genuine interaction. Being "real" or genuine grounds the basic elements of healing conversation: listening carefully and responding thoughtfully. Indeed, a genuine conversation is possible only in the company of people who are open to the experience of the other. This sentiment was captured with great wisdom by philosopher Hans Gadamer: "Thus a genuine conversation is never the one we wanted to conduct."[4] It is always the product of the interaction of two people, individual agendas joined in genuine openness to the other's agenda.

2. Presence

Presence is the ability to be with another person emotionally and physically. It may sound simple, but it is particularly difficult when external distractions (a busy household, active children) or internal distractions (anxiety, thinking about what to say) intrude. Being present does not mean absorbing another's emotions or collapsing under the weight of another's pain. The "fusion delusion," where one person is so wrapped up in another's emotions that he or she loses track of his or her own, muddies the water and only confuses people in mortal time. Being present without taking over another's pain or projecting one's own feelings onto another is a complicated, delicate dance.

Sometimes presence with boundaries proves impossible for a family member, so close to a loved one that he or she can sense every emotion. Presence also involves physically attending to another. By "attending," we simply mean looking at and listening to a conversation partner. Being emotionally, physically, and psychologically present can be profoundly healing in and of itself even without words. In conversation, this is often as simple as following the lead of the other by putting one's own conversational agenda on the back burner. Being at the side of a loved one for doctor's appointments or sitting quietly at the bedside in the hospital are opportunities to provide powerful presence. The essence of presence is being there for the other, putting his or her needs first. Strong presence is not easily achieved. Not many of us are accustomed to suspending our needs and paying attention to another in an intense way for long periods of time.

3. *Sensitivity*

Sensitivity refers to the awareness of the emotional state and needs of others and oneself. This state requires "people reading" skills—the ability to look at a person and make some accurate judgment as to what he or she might be feeling given his or her body language, voice tone, pace of speech, and any other cues. It is always risky to assume you know what someone is feeling, even though body language can provide clues. Some people seem to have a knack for it. It is important that the person who is attempting to understand and be sensitive to the other not assume that he or she "knows what the other person is really feeling." Tentativeness is golden here. For example, "You seem sad today. Are you feeling down?" is a gentle challenge and invitation to recognize underlying feelings that may be more or less in one's awareness. Sensitivity also involves being aware of one's own feelings so as not to confuse them with the feelings of another. It is all too easy to assume mistakenly that we understand the experience of another person, particularly for professional caregivers who have been in mortal time with many people over many years. No two people experience mortal time in quite the same way, and one of the challenges is to maintain sensitivity to the unique responses of each individual.

4. Courage

Courage is required to accompany another in mortal time. It is the mental and moral strength to persevere in the face of danger and difficulty. The diagnosis of grave illness presents patients and their loved ones with an immediate threat to their way of life and often a difficult path ahead through treatment and follow-up care. Courage is a quality that can be cultivated through conversations in mortal time. Companions may accompany their loved ones through repeated doctor appointments and difficult test procedures that can shake even sturdy resolve. Particularly distressing are the moments when outcomes of lab tests or scans are not good. The news that a patient did not do well in chemotherapy is often made bearable only by the presence of a fellow traveler, a companion in mortal time. In order to be there and stay there, companions must be able to tolerate this and many other distressing situations, like waiting for long periods of time to see doctors, missing work, and foregoing travel and normal leisure pursuits. A normal schedule becomes a thing of the past as the demands of faithful companionship in mortal time take over, calling for the quality of courage.

5. Acceptance

Acceptance of another's illness and the demanding path that it may put one on is no simple task. For starters, it requires time simply to absorb the reality of life-threatening circumstances. We want to underscore that acceptance is not giving up, but may mean letting go of the effort to control a situation fraught with ambiguity and uncertainties. This requires wisdom, and it is no simple matter to know when it is time to accept a situation rather than try to change it. Acceptance may bring a profound sense of peace. The disposition of acceptance is classically expressed in this excerpt from the "Serenity Prayer" of the late theologian Reinhold Niebuhr:

> God grant me the serenity to accept the things I cannot change; the courage to change the things I can; and the wisdom to know the difference.

6. *Respect*

Respect signals our appreciation of the dignity and worth of another. It is communicated by both what we say and how we act toward a person. The opposite of respectful conversation is often seen in today's "talk" shows where commentators routinely attempt to prove their intellectual superiority by shouting or arguing down others. Respect in conversation requires thoughtful, patient listening, responding with care and sometimes with deference to the other's personal circumstances. Respectful communication is ordinarily characterized by give and take. For physicians and nurses this includes giving simple and clear explanations of complex medical facts to patients and family members unfamiliar with the language of medicine. Doing so respectfully requires awareness of where the patient is starting from and understanding of the situation from the patient's perspective. The task is made more difficult by a fact that we noted earlier: a once-in-a-lifetime experience for the patient is an everyday event for the medical practitioner. The medical person may be hard pressed to be patient when answering the same question for the fifth time that day, albeit from a different person. Often the same question is repeated by a single patient because the answer already given is startling and not comprehensible, even when it was put in simple language. In such moments, companions must strive to remember that what a person is really absorbing is not information, but mortality. An exhausted, exasperated caregiver may end up talking in a patronizing manner. Even when unintended, this is not an ingredient of respectful interaction. Recognizing and embracing mortal time is a life-long process that dawns slowly in the natural aging process as the physical and mental losses slowly accumulate with human wear and tear. This process is often accelerated under the press of life-threatening illness.

7. Compassion

Compassion for another involves understanding what someone is experiencing, especially his or her circumstances and suffering. This can be both powerful and painful, as anyone who has held a sobbing loved one knows. Compassion is the virtue that drives empathy, which we discussed at length in Part II. Compassionate caregivers are at some risk of getting overwhelmed by the suffering of the one who is ill. For example, the diagnosis of a life-threatening illness such as cancer often renders a person numb and stunned. A loved one sitting with him or her as the diagnosis is communicated will likely experience similar feelings, and yet it is important for him or her to be able to function so as to help the other cope. Strong presence in the form of a touch of the arm, holding hands, or another appropriate physical gesture as well as a pledge to "stick with you in this" from the companion can be very reassuring in these circumstances.

Patients experience the compassion of their professional and family caregivers through many gestures such as a hug or what we call "kind eyes." To look on another's suffering with kind eyes is to take that suffering into one's heart and hold it there gently. For the family caregiver experiencing his or her own pain as well, this can be very difficult, perhaps impossible, initially. The caregiver's distress, as well as that of his or her loved one, calls for comfort, posing an even more formidable challenge for medical personnel. Health-care providers themselves may become numbed to suffering and indeed may need to be shielded from the sheer volume of distress pumped into their worlds each day. Imagine the challenge of being compassionate to 20 or 30 patients and family members facing life-threatening circumstances each day! Compassionate caregivers must find sources to nourish themselves. Paradoxically, one source of compassion can be the very patients and families who need their care.

8. Humor

Humor is a saving grace in mortal time, as in all of life. People facing frightening circumstances cannot sustain the energy necessary to stay frightened over long periods. They need relief from tension. Humor can be profoundly healing in times of intense distress but must be used tactfully since it can backfire and send a message of disrespect. Knowing a person's sensibilities is important here, because what evokes laughter in one person might cause acute pain for another. This is a place where it is important to follow the lead of the other. Sometimes a person's sense of humor in these circumstances can be striking. People cry and laugh even in the midst of horrendous suffering, fear, and distress. There can be healthy forms of expressing humor as well as maladaptive ones, where humor appears to be masking deep sorrow, in the effort to stave off grieving that might be necessary for acceptance.

A patient illustrated his own appreciation for irony and a good sense of humor when he reflected, "It's amazing how nice people are to you when they think you're going to die." He had recently undergone a life-threatening treatment, returned home safely, and was remembering how friends and relatives treated him after his initial diagnosis, when it was felt that there was little that medical treatment could offer him and before he traveled across the country to Seattle for a life-saving and risky bone marrow transplant. This is an excellent example of the saving grace of a sense of humor. He was able to laugh at his own peculiar circumstances, at how he saw others seeing him.

Healing can occur when humor and laughter enter mortal-time conversation, sometimes in very unusual ways. So- called "gallows humor" can lighten the burden of both patient and caregiver. One patient joked, "I won't have to worry about paying my life insurance premiums any more!" This type of humor has risks and is best initiated by the patient rather than the caregiver. An example of a statement that could be hurtful is the following, overheard in a busy cancer clinic: "Are you still alive?" A professional caregiver asked that question of a patient who he had not seen in a long time. The patient and professional both laughed heartily and began a brief conversation. This appeared to go over well because the question was posed in a joking manner. However, one can see how this might be upsetting to a patient and linger on in the imagination in the form of questions such as, "I wonder what he meant by that; does he expect me to die soon?" Humor, like fire, can warm—or burn.

9. *Awareness of limitations*

Finally, the caregiver who is a family member of a loved one or a professional working with patients daily must come to some *awareness of personal limitations*. The caregiver cannot take all the pain away when life-threatening illness arrives. One who loves or cares for another will suffer when they do. We cannot spare our loved ones or patients the sorrow and pain that is a part of each and every one of our lives. This may be the most difficult reality of the hard lessons in being a faithful companion in mortal time—we are limited in our ability to protect those for whom we care from suffering.

Every caregiver companion has physical and emotional limitations. Knowing when the limits of physical endurance are reached will help caregivers avoid complete exhaustion. We have seen professional and family companions push the limits of endurance and make themselves sick. A wise companion learns when to stop and take a break in order to do the good work of caregiving. In our next sections we address the following question often asked of caregivers, both family and professional: How can you do this, anyway?

A WORD TO CAREGIVERS
"How can you do this, anyway?"

This question is often asked of professional caregivers by patients, family members, and those unfamiliar with the challenge and promise of mortal time. It is also a question for anybody who is a caregiver of a seriously ill family member, a likely role for all of us at one time or another. One answer is that meeting others with compassion and honesty in mortal time has many intrinsic rewards, including a deep satisfaction at helping others, which increases our own capacity to love. Caring for another may in fact be a gift to oneself, a pouring out of one's own cup of caring that can, paradoxically, fill it back up. Giving becomes receiving.

RESILIENCE AND ABSORBING SUFFERING

As we have said, once-in-a-lifetime, shattering events for patients and their families and friends are "normal" for a professional caregiver. How can a person be repeatedly exposed to the shocking entrance into mortal time without becoming depressed or unglued? Traveling regularly on the ground of mortal time requires and develops two personal qualities. The first is psychological resilience, which is the capacity to adapt well in the face of adversity. A serious life-threatening illness will tax anyone, and being resilient does not mean that no emotional distress will be experienced. On the contrary, emotional pain and suffering are inevitable, even for the resilient person. Resilience is not a quality that people either have or not. We all have some capacity to be resilient, and what we have can be deepened intentionally. Resilience can develop out of repeated experience with adversity. However, some people seem to develop this capacity more deeply than others. One quality of resilient people is the ability to manage strong feelings and impulses. We know a physician who has a custom of taking a deep breath and offering a short prayer before entering the exam room of her next cancer patient, thereby restoring herself from her previous encounter and preparing herself for her next. This is just one example of a simple, practical way to remain effective and resilient in a hectic clinic full of patients and caregivers managing their lives in mortal time.

The second quality necessary for traveling in mortal time is the capacity to absorb suffering without becoming overwhelmed by it. Some have referred to this as establishing psychological boundaries, so that at the end of the day the professional caregiver can go home and, for the most part, leave the suffering behind. But what professional caregiver doesn't periodically lie awake at night, troubled by his or her patient's struggle? Of course, the family caregiver, particularly the primary caregiver, is more exposed and will be unable to leave his or her situation behind as professional caregivers do every day.

EMPATHY SHIFT

What is the down side to daily exposure to the rigors of mortal time? Can spending day after day in the company of suffering affect a caregiver's emotional sensibility? Yes. Seeing and being with those subjected to suffering has a profound impact on a caregiver's perception. Some may

One cannot enter conversation about mortal time with an open heart and remain untouched. It hurts to encounter the suffering of another. However, healing and helping in the midst of suffering is an altruistic act and can be its own reward. We can become "larger" when we listen and empathize with the life story of another. Bernard Loomer describes this phenomenon figuratively as "growing in stature": our soul expands in size.[5] This happens whenever we compassionately take in the life experience of another person, in this case the suffering of a person struggling in mortal time.

experience a change in the ability to empathize with the normal and expected small wounds of everyday life. After being confronted with the stark pain and disruption of cancer, how is one to respond to a 15-year-old whose shoes don't quite match the color of her prom dress? Or the cold and flu-like symptoms of a spouse? As a colleague so aptly puts it, "It takes a lot more to get my attention—if it isn't cancer, just get over it." If, as we suggested in Part II, empathy is the capacity to "walk in another's shoes," chronic exposure to severe health problems may limit the caregiver's ability to relate empathically with a person experiencing everyday non-life-threatening health problems. The caregiver's empathy threshold shifts such that a distressful event experienced by someone has to be a lot more serious in order to reach the point where it triggers an empathic response. Another's suffering may need to be acute and related to a significant stressor to activate the ability of the professional caregiver to respond empathically. The phenomenon of diminished empathy, or empathy shift, can have major implications for the day-to-day communication of caregivers with those outside their personal or professional "kingdom of suffering." One antidote to the negative effects of empathy shift is to take breaks from repeated exposure to deep suffering in mortal time. Another is to talk about suffering with a friend or colleague who has the ability to listen carefully and respond thoughtfully.

SHARING THE DARKNESS

Conversation in mortal time exposes both the caregiver and the person who may be dying to powerful psychological forces. Two metaphors can illuminate these forces. The first, described by physician Sheila Cassidy, concerns darkness. Dr. Cassidy calls the experience of suffering with another "sharing the darkness."[6] The caregiver proceeding into mortal time with another does so at personal risk, for in sharing the darkness, one cannot help but absorb some of it into one's soul. In a real conversation with one who is awake in mortal time, the most healthy and psychologically resilient caregiver will experience this darkening as he or she loses the comforting but false presumption of time's endlessness. Encountering death is not for the faint of heart, but, paradoxically, strength does not lie in stoic, unemotional encounter but rather in awareness and acceptance of one's own emotional responses, including intense anxiety. In the deepening shade of mortal time, as they encounter vicariously the prospect of their own deaths, caregivers can begin to see their own lives with clear vision.

MENDING

The second metaphor comes from the C. K. Williams poem entitled "Invisible Mending."[7] In the poem, Williams depicts three old women, sewing and using "their amputating shears: forgiveness and repair." He compares sewing garments with the tasks of forgiveness and repair that necessarily accompany all human relating. The emotional healing that occurs in conversation in mortal time is a form of invisible mending. This image is also captured in the Jewish conception of the human vocation—*tikkun olam*—to bind up the world's brokenness.

THE ART OF CONVERSATION THROUGH SERIOUS ILLNESS

The transformative possibility embedded in the experience of mortal time derives from facing death as the potential limit of all human existence. This disturbing possibility in turn carries the blessed opportunity to consider one's life, make amends where possible, and say what is in one's heart to family, friends, and associates—to finish one's life with deliberateness and a measure of closure denied to those who die suddenly or who "successfully" evade the awareness of mortality.

The claim we make in these pages is simple, but never easy to honor: Whatever the details of a life-threatening illness, and however great the differences in backgrounds, roles, and responsibilities of those communicating about it, authentic conversation has the power to enhance how people cope with living in mortal time. Real talking and listening can illuminate and enrich the very meaning of life for those caregivers and people living in this sacred place together. The liberating possibility embedded in the experience of mortal time is the freedom that can come from facing death squarely as the limit of our existence. We must embrace what we mortals fear and ordinarily avoid with every fiber of our being. We must turn toward death together, in a shared movement that opens into life-giving possibility.

NOTES

PROLOGUE

1. "On Earth," from *Walking to Martha's Vineyard* (New York: Knopf, 2003), 4, by Franz Wright, copyright © by Franz Wright. Used by permission of Alfred A. Knopf, a division of Random House, Inc.

INTRODUCTION

1. Parts of this book have appeared in two previously published articles: M. A. Cowan and R. P. McQuellon, "Turning toward death together," *The Furrow* (July/August 2000): 395–402; and R. P. McQuellon and M. A. Cowan, "Turning toward death together: Conversation in mortal time," *The American Journal of Hospice & Palliative Care* 17 (2000): 9, 312–318.

2. M. Lerner, *Choices in Healing: Integrating the Best of Conventional and Complementary Approaches to Cancer* (Cambridge, MA: MIT Press, 1996), xix.

PART I

THE MANY MEANINGS OF MORTAL TIME

1. The lines reproduced here are from Theodore Roethke's poem "In a Dark Time," which appears in *The Collected Poems of Theodore Roethke* (New York: Doubleday, 1966), 231.

2. We are indebted to Barbara Sourkes and her explication of the concept "neutral time." See B. Sourkes, *The Deepening Shade: Psychological Aspects of Life-Threatening Illness* (Pittsburg: University of Pittsburg Press, 1982). Dr. Sourkes acknowledges Margaret Clare Kiely, who coined the term "neutral time" to capture the experience of patients who enter this "living-dying interval."

3. Life expectancy is the average period that a person may expect to live. A life expectancy table lists how long an individual might expect to live, given his or her current age. For example, a 60-year-old man might expect live another 22 years barring an unpredictable accident. Insurance companies and benefit planners use these tables to calculate premiums for health insurance and what funds might be needed for retirement, given an expected life span.

4. James and Evelyn Whitehead. *Method in Ministry*. (New York: Seabury Press, 1980), 149–151.

5. Jerome D. Frank, *Persuasion and Healing: A Comparative Study of Psychotherapy* (Rev. Ed.) (Baltimore: Johns Hopkins University Press, 1973).

6. R. Janoff-Bulman, *Shattered Assumptions: Toward a Psychology of Trauma* (New York: Free Press, 1992).

7. Faust, D. G. *This Republic of Suffering: Death and the American Civil War.* (New York: Alfred A. Knopf, 2008).

8. D. F. Cella, "Health promotion in oncology: A cancer wellness doctrine," *Journal of Psychosocial Oncology* 8 (1990): 1, 17–31.

9. C. M. Orsborn et al., *Speak the Language of Healing: Living with Breast Cancer Without Going to War* (Berkeley: Conari Press, 1989).

10. Dr. Chip Celestino is the course director of the Dr.-Patient relationship course at Wake Forest University School of Medicine. First-year medical students are placed in groups of four to five students with two faculty members for 33 total contact hours. There is a series of readings and a text that address topics such as developing rapport, using empathy, respecting diversity, the difficult patient, etc. Each student conducts six or more observed interviews with hospitalized patients, interviews with three to four standardized patients, and role play various scenarios, e.g., giving bad news. Nearly all activities are directly observed by faculty who provide immediate feedback.

11. A. Ornstein, "The dread to repeat," *Journal of the American Psychoanalytic Association* 39 (1989): 377–398.

12. C. Geertz, *The Interpretation of Cultures* (New York: Basic Books, 1973), 100–108.

13. M. Heidegger, *Being and Time,* trans. J. Stambaugh (Albany: SUNY Press, 1996).

14. Cited in E. T. Chambers and M. A. Cowan, *Roots for Radicals* (New York: Continuum, 2005), 59.

15. H. Sigler, *Hollis Sigler's Breast Cancer Journal* (New York: Hudson Hills Press, 1999).

16. J. Kabat-Zinn, *Wherever You Go, There You Are: Mindfulness Meditation in Everyday Life* (New York: Hyperion Books, 1994).

17. Personal communication between Bob Stone and Richard McQuellon, January 15, 1993. Also, see Bob Stone and Jenny Stone Humphries, *Where the Buffaloes Roam: Building a Team for Life's Challenges* (Boston: Addison Wesley Publishing Company, 1993).

18. R. G. Smith, *Martin Buber* (Richmond: John Knox Press, 1967), 14.

PART II

HOPE FROM CONVERSATION

1. G. Marcel, *Tragic Wisdom and Beyond* (Evanston: Northwestern University Press, 1973), 143.

2. V. Havel, *Disturbing the Peace: A Conversation with Karel Huizdala* (New York: Random House, 1991), 199.

3. Stephen Jay Gould, "The Median Isn't the Message," *Steve Dunn's CancerGuide*, http://cancerguide.org/median_not_msg.html (26 August 2007).

4. A. Broyard, *Intoxicated by My Illness: And Other Writings on Life and Death* (New York: Crown Publishers: 1992).

5. L. A. Fogarty, B. A. Curbow, J. R. Wingard, K. McDonnell, and M. R. Somerfield, "Can 40 seconds of compassion reduce patient anxiety?" *Journal of Clinical Oncology* 17 (1999): 1, 371–379.

6. Ephesians 4:15, *The New Oxford Annotated Bible* (New York: Oxford University Press, 1991).

7. William Shakespeare, *Julius Caesar* 2.2.32–34, in *The Complete Works of William Shakespeare* (Roslyn, NY: Walter J. Black, 1937), 870.

8. J. Rieveschl and M. Cowan, *Selfhood and the Dance of Empathy. Progress in Self Psychology*, vol. 19 (Hillsdale, NJ: The Analytic Press, 2003), 107–132.

9. Nina Ann Stokes was a courageous volunteer, colleague, and breast cancer patient who managed her diagnosis and many recurrences and treatments with grace and determination. She was an inspiration to members of the Cancer Patient Support Program community. She died on March 14, 2001, nine years after her initial diagnosis. After one of her many treatments, she developed peripheral neuropathy. Peripheral neuropathy is a condition caused by damage to the nerves in the peripheral nervous system. Many of these nerves are involved with sensation and feeling things such as pain, temperature, and touch. Peripheral neuropathy is usually felt at

first as tingling and numbness in the hands and feet. Symptoms can be described as burning, shooting pain, throbbing, aching, and "feels like frostbite" or "walking on a bed of coals." It is most commonly a side effect of some drugs used to treat cancer.

10. W. I. Thomas and D. S. Thomas, *The Child in America* (NY: Knopf, 1928), 572.

11. E. Fox, K. Landrum-McNiff, Z. Zhong, N. V. Dawson, A. W. Wu, and J. Lynn, "Evaluation of prognostic criteria for determining hospice eligibility in patients with advanced lung, heart, or liver cancer," *JAMA* 282 (1999): 1638–1645. This study points out that some chronically ill patients may "never experience a time during which they are clearly dying of their disease." By "clearly dying" the authors are referring to acute symptoms that are imminently life threatening. Predicting the length of remaining life probably is best done on the following continuum: hours to days, days to weeks, weeks to months, and months to years. Indeed, some hospice patients graduate to home rather than the graveyard.

12. Anton Chekhov, "Misery—To Whom Shall I Tell My Grief?" in *Anton Chekhov's Short Stories*, ed. Ralph E. Maitlaw (New York: W.W. Norton & Co., 1979), 11–16.

13. C. L. Loprinzi, M. E. Johnson, and G. Steer, "Doc, how much time do I have?" *Journal of Clinical Oncology* 18 (2000) 3, 699–701.

14. D. G. Larson and D. R. Tobin, "End of life conversations: evolving practice and theory," *JAMA* 284 (2000):12, 1573–1578.

PART III

GUIDANCE FOR CAREGIVERS

1. Ecclesiastes 3:1, *The New Oxford Annotated Bible* (New York: Oxford University Press, 1991).

2. L. G. Calhoun and R. G. Tedeschi, "Expert companions: Posttraumatic growth in clinical practice," in *Handbook of Posttraumatic Growth*, eds. Calhoun and Tedeschi (Mahwah, NJ: Lawrence Erlbaum Associates, Inc., 2006).

3. We are grateful to Dr. Richard Tedeschi for his thoughtful explanation of some of the qualities necessary for expert companioning in a lecture he gave at the Wake Forest University Baptist Medical Center Comprehensive Cancer Center, September 1, 2006.

4. Gadamer, H. G. *Truth and Method.* 2nd rev. edition. Trans. J. Weinsheimer and D. G. Marshall. New York: Crossroad, 1989.

5. B. Loomer, "S-I-Z-E is the measure," in *Religious Experience and Process Theology*, eds. H. Cargas and B. Lee (NY: Paulist Press, 1976) 69–76.

6. S. Cassidy, *Sharing the Darkness: The Spirituality of Caring* (Marynoll, NY: Orbis Books, 1991). In her fine work, Dr. Cassidy quotes Anglican author J. B. Phillips. Suffering from deep depression, Phillips "shared this darkness" with a colleague, noting, "There is no way out, only a way forward."

7. C. K. Williams, *Repair* (New York: Farrar, Straus and Giroux, 1999).

BIBLIOGRAPHY

Broyard, A. *Intoxicated by My Illness: And Other Writings on Life and Death.* New York: Crown Publishers, 1992.

Calhoun, L. G., and R. G. Tedeschi. "Expert companions: Posttraumatic growth in clinical practice." In *Handbook of Posttraumatic Growth.* Edited by Calhoun and Tedeschi. Mahwah, NJ: Lawrence Erlbaum Associates, Inc., 2006.

Cassidy, S. *Sharing the Darkness: The Spirituality of Caring.* Marynoll, NY: Orbis Books, 1991.

Cella, D. F. "Health promotion in oncology: A cancer wellness doctrine." *Journal of Psychosocial Oncology* 8 (1990): 1, 17–31.

Chambers, E. T., and M. A. Cowan, *Roots for Radicals.* New York: Continuum, 2005.

Chekhov, A. "Misery—To Whom Shall I Tell My Grief?" In *Anton Chekhov's Short Stories.* Edited by Ralph E. Maitlaw, 11–16. New York: W. W. Norton & Co., 1979.

Cowan, M. A., and R. P. McQuellon. "Turning toward death together." *The Furrow* (July/August 2000): 395–402.

Fogarty, L. A., B. A. Curbow, J. R. Wingard, K. McDonnell, and M. R. Somerfield. "Can 40 seconds of compassion reduce patient anxiety?" *Journal of Clinical Oncology* 17 (1999): 1, 371–379.

Fox, E., K. Landrum-McNiff, Z. Zhong, N. V. Dawson, A. W. Wu, and J. Lynn. "Evaluation of prognostic criteria for determining hospice eligibility in patients with advanced lung, heart, or liver cancer." *JAMA* 282 (1999): 1638–1645.

Frank, J. D., *Persuasion and Healing: A Comparative Study of Psychotherapy.* (Rev. Ed.) Baltimore: Johns Hopkins University Press, 1973.

Gadamer, H. G. *Truth and Method.* 2nd rev. edition. Trans. J. Weinsheimer and D. G. Marshall. New York: Crossroad, 1989.

Geertz, C. *The Interpretation of Cultures.* New York: Basic Books, 1973.

Gilpin Faust, D. *This Republic of Suffering: Death and the American Civil War.* New York: Alfred A. Knopf, 2008.

Gould, S. J. "The Median Isn't the Message." *Steve Dunn's Cancer Guide.* http://cancerguide.org/median_not_msg.html.

Havel, V. *Disturbing the Peace: A Conversation with Karel Huizdala.* New York: Random House, 1991.

Heidegger, M. *Being and Time.* Translated by J. Stambaugh. Albany: SUNY Press, 1996.

Janoff-Bulman, R. *Shattered Assumptions: Toward a Psychology of Trauma.* New York: Free Press, 1992.

Kabat-Zinn, J. *Wherever You Go, There You Are: Mindfulness Meditation in Everyday Life.* New York: Hyperion Books, 1994.

Larson, D. G., and D. R. Tobin. "End of life conversations: evolving practice and theory." *JAMA* 284 (2000): 12, 1573–1578.

Lerner M. *Choices in Healing: Integrating the Best of Conventional and Complementary Approaches to Cancer.* Cambridge, MA: MIT Press, 1996.

Loomer, B. "S-I-Z-E is the measure." In *Religious Experience and Process Theology.* Edited by H. Cargas and B. Lee, 69–76. NY: Paulist Press, 1976.

Loprinzi, C. L., M. E. Johnson, and G. Steer. "Doc, how much time do I have?" *Journal of Clinical Oncology* 18 (2000): 3, 699–701.

Marcel, G. *Tragic Wisdom and Beyond.* Evanston: Northwestern University Press, 1973.

McQuellon, R. P., and M. A. Cowan. "Turning toward death together: Conversation in mortal time." *The American Journal of Hospice & Palliative Care* 17 (2000): 9, 312–318.

The New Oxford Annotated Bible. New York: Oxford University Press, 1991.

Ornstein A. "The dread to repeat." *Journal of the American Psychoanalytic Association* 39 (1989): 377–398.

Orsborn, C. M., L. Quigley, K. L. Stroup, and S. Kuner. *Speak the Language of Healing: Living with Breast Cancer Without Going to War.* Berkeley: Conari Press, 1989.

Rieveschl, J., and M. Cowan. *Selfhood and the Dance of Empathy. Progress in Self Psychology.* Vol. 19. Hillsdale, NJ: The Analytic Press, 2003.

Roethke, T. "In a Dark Time." In *The Collected Poems of Theodore Roethke,* 231. New York: Doubleday, 1966.

Shakespeare, W. *Julius Caesar.* In *The Complete Works of William Shakespeare,* 860–888. Roslyn, NY: Walter J. Black, 1937.

Sigler, H. *Hollis Sigler's Breast Cancer Journal.* New York: Hudson Hills Press, 1999.

Smith, R. G. *Martin Buber.* Richmond: John Knox Press, 1967.

Sourkes, B. *The Deepening Shade: Psychological Aspects of Life-Threatening Illness.* Pittsburg: University of Pittsburg Press, 1982.

Stone, B., and J. S. Humphries. *Where the Buffaloes Roam: Building a Team for Life's Challenges.* Boston: Addison Wesley Publishing Company, 1993.

Thomas, W. I., and D. S. Thomas. *The Child in America.* NY: Knopf, 1928.

Williams, C. K. *Repair.* New York: Farrar, Straus and Giroux, 1999.

Wright, F. "On Earth." In *Walking to Martha's Vineyard,* 4. New York: Knopf, 2003.

INDEX

Acceptance, 110–11
American culture
    denial and, 89
    dying and, 7
Anger, while living in mortal time, 42
Anxiety
    death, 105
    management of, 104–5
Assumptive world
    coping styles reflected from,
        20–24
    life events influencing, 17–18
    mortal time and, 17–18
    spiritual belief and, 18
Authentic conversation and, 124
    despair and, 36
    living authentically, 38
Awkwardness
    of death talk, 95
    of mortal time, 15–16, 83

Benevolence, of world, 19
Birth's possibility, 3
Breast Cancer Journal (Sigler, Hollis), 39
Broyard, Anatole, 54
Buber, Martin, 45

"Burden shared is but half a
        trouble", 63

Caregiver(s). *See also* Professional
        caregivers
    anxiety management and, 104–5
    challenge for, 104
    compassion and, 104
    definition of, 8
    diagnosis and, 15
    fear and, 74
    guidance for, 8–9, 99–124
    mortal time and, 49–50
    personal limitation awareness of,
        116–17
    silence of, 69–70
Cassidy, Sheila, 122
Cella, David, 20, 21
Chatter, everyday, 88–89
Chekhov, Anton, 76
"Click of contact," 54–55
Communication
    compassionate, 87
    failure of, 27
    nonverbal, 55–56
    training in, 27

Companion(s)
    kind, 100–104
    mortal time and, 99–100
    schedule alteration and, 102–3
    support/self-care from, 105
    types of, 99
Companionship
    costs/risks of, 104–5
    family dynamics and, 103
    needed during mortal time, 62
    suffering and, 104
Compassion, 113–14
    caregivers and, 104
    "compassion fatigue", 105
    gestures of, 114
    mortality posture on, 40
    powerful/painful, 113
    professional caregivers and, 114
Compassionate conversation, 87
Conversation, 54–56. See also Healing
        conversation
    censored v. active listening, 85–86
    compassionate, 87
    consideration/disciplined
        spontaneity in, 82–85
    death talk v. life talk, 93–94
    about dying, 92–94
    everyday chatter and, 88–89
    with friends, 75–77

genuineness and, 107
heavy v. light, 88
honesty in, 58–59, 70–72
"how much time do I have?",
    87–88
metaphors and, 94
mutual acknowledgment and, 55
partners of, 62–63
platitudes and, 77–80
practical, 94–95
respect in, 111–12
silence and, 71
Coping styles
    assumptive worlds reflection on,
        20–24
    combination of, 20–21
    fighters and, 23
    for mortal time, 20–24
    opportunists and, 22
    peacemakers and, 24
    pessimists and, 21
    realists and, 21
    zealots and, 22–23
Courage, 109–10

Daily activities, 41
Death
    character/significance of, 38
    confrontation of, 13, 31–33

dealing with possibility of, 5
emotions arising from, 9
feelings/behavior shaped by, 5
"giving up" and, 60
impending, hope and, 35
preoccupation fluctuation of, 28
preoccupation with, 27–29
prospect of, 29, 94
receptivity to, 40–41
Death anxiety, 105
Death talk, 7
awkwardness/sensitivity of, 95
life talk v., 93–94
Denial, 89–92
American culture and, 89
avoidance and, 91
importance/usefulness of, 91
Depression, 34–35
Despair
depression and, 34–35
hope balance with, 34
prospect of, 35–37
suicide and, 34–35
Diagnosis. See also Life-threatening
diagnosis
calmness during, 5
caregivers and, 15
language and, 26–27
as shocking/stunning, 26–27

Dying
American culture and, 7
healthy conversation about, 92–94
preoccupation with, 7
total focus on, 28

Empathy, 57
becoming properly, 66–68
for unknown experiences, 66–67
growing in stature and, 120
hope and, 63
information and, 74
is a quality and specific behavior, 64
listening and, 67
platitudes and, 76
power of, 64–65
quality of, 66
receiving of, 68–70
self-reflection/self-examination
for, 66
two steps for, 64
understanding and, 57
Empathy shift
antidote for, 121–22
of professional caregivers, 120–22
threshold of, 121

False hope, 35, 53–54
Family dynamics, 103

Fear
    acknowledgment of, 73–75
    caregivers and, 74
    mortal time and, 65
"The feared future dominating the
    lived present," 28
Feelings
    death's shape of, 5
    expression of, 57
    healing conversation and, 57
    management of, 119
Fighters, 23
"Foot in mouth" syndrome, 84
Frank, Jerome, 16
Friends
    conversations with, 75–77
    normal behavior of, 75
"Fusion delusion," 107
Future, hoped-for, loss of, 25–26

Gadamer, Hans, 107
"Gallows humor," 116
Geertz, Clifford, 36
Genuineness, 106–7
"Giving up," 60
Gloom avoidance, 52–53
Goals, needed for hope,
    51–52
Gould, Stephen Jay, 54

Havel, Vaclav, 50
Healing conversation, 55
    basic elements of, 56–59
    feelings and, 57
    invitation to, 61
    listening and, 57–58
    personal assumptions and, 56–57
    requirements for, 57–58
    thoughtful/honest response and,
        58–59
Heidegger, Martin, 38
Honesty, 58–59
    fact and truth and, 71
    in conversation, 58–59, 70–72
    needed for hope, 63
    professional caregivers and, 71
    right words and, 72
    suffering and, 73
    words well spoken and, 71
Hope
    abrupt removal of, 51
    for the day, 49–52
    despair balance with, 34
    empathy/honesty needed for, 63
    false, 35, 53–54
    goals needed for, 51–52
    Havel on, 50
    impending death and, 35
    maintaining/losing, 50

Marcel on, 50
from mortal time, 21
sources of, 39, 44–45
spiritual belief and, 45
"How much time do I have?", 87–88
Humor
    "gallows," 116
    healthy/maladaptive expression
        forms of, 115
    tension release from, 114

Insensitivity, of professional
        caregivers, 26–27, 84–85
Intrusive thoughts, 28, 42
"Invisible Mending" (Williams, C.K.),
        123
"Is this all there is?", 34

Janoff-Bulman, Ronnie, 18

Kabat-Zinn, Jon, 42
"Kairos" time, 15
"Kind eyes," 114

Language, for diagnosis, 26–27
    "dosing" and, 80
Lerner, Michael, 6
Life events/-style
    assumptive world influenced by,
        17–18

life-threatening diagnosis changes
        to, 32–33
Life span, losses experienced in, 30
Life-threatening diagnosis, 6, 27
    confrontation of, 8
    lifestyle changes from, 32–33
    role changes due to, 30
    as shattering experience, 20
"Life will go on" assumption, 29
Listening
    acknowledgement and, 75
    active v. censored conversation,
        85–86
    carefully and respond
        thoughtfully, 6, 50, 57–58, 75, 82,
        107, 122
    empathy and, 67
    healing conversations and, 57–58
Living
    authentically, 38
    gracefully, 5–6
    with mortality, 5–7
    in mortal time, 41–44
Loomer, Bernard, 120

Marcel, Gabriel, 50
Meaning
    creation of, 19–46
    from events, 19

Meaning (*Continued*)
  existence of, 45–46
  finding, 37–41
  in interpreter's mind, 19
Meaningfulness, of world, 19
Meaninglessness, 34
Meaning-of-life
  questions, 33–34, 105
  threat for, 36–38
"The Median Isn't the Message"
  (Gould, Stephen, Jay), 54
Medical providers. *See* Professional
  caregivers
"Misery—To Whom Shall I Tell My
  Grief?" (Chekhov, Anton), 76
Mortality
  compassionate/receptive/
    reflective posture on, 40
  consideration of, 29
  embracing of, 7
  living with, 5–7
  median, 54
  obsession on, 4
  promise and despair and, 39
  realities of, 15
  trivialization of, 3–4
Mortal time, 6, 13–46
  assumptive world and, 17–18
  awkwardness of, 15–16, 83
  blessings of, 123–24
  caregivers and, 49–50
  challenge/invitation of, 33–34
  companions and, 99–100
  companionship needed during, 62
  coping skills for, 20–24
  daily activities and, 41
  death confrontation and, 13, 31–33
  effective phrases in, 81–82
  emotional balance of, 88
  entry into, 24–27, 49
  expectations of, 24–33
  fear and, 65
  grief of development and, 30
  hope from, 21
  "how to be" in, 7
  intrusive thoughts and, 28, 42
  as "kairos" time, 15
  length of, 14–18, 43
  life-long embracing process of,
    112–13
  living authentically due to, 38
  living in, 41–44
  loss of words and, 71
  meaning found by, 37–41
  multiple meanings of, 16–18
  paradox of, 39, 42–43
  personal assumptions shattered by,
    43–44

personal history influencing, 16
sense of loss and, 29–31
sense of urgency from, 32
spiritual tradition and, 16–17
talking in/about, 59–61
treatment during, 14
virtues most needed in,
106–17
Mortal time experience
as changing, 31–33
direct/acute, 13, 42–43
as personal, 15, 29
as shattering, 20
as vicarious, 13

Niebuhr, Reinhold, 111
Nonverbal communication,
professional caregivers and,
55–56

Opportunists, 22
Ornstein, Anna, 34
Orsborn, Carol, 24

Peacemakers, 24
Personal assumptions
healing conversations and,
56–57
mortal time shattering, 43–44

Personal limitation awareness
of caregivers, 116–17
physical/emotional, 117
Pessimists, 21
Platitudes, 77–80
common phrases of, 78–79
empathy and, 76
harm done from, 80
as insult, 70
ritualized quality of, 77
"you first", 80–81
Practical conversation, 94–95
Presence, 107–8
boundaries and, 108
difficult task of, 103
"fusion delusion" and, 107
internal/external distractions
to, 107
Professional caregivers
compassion and, 114
empathy shift of, 120–22
encouragement from, 62
honesty and, 71
"how much time do I have?"
conversation and, 87–88
insensitivity/tactlessness of,
26–27, 84–85
intrinsic rewards for, 118
mending of, 123

Professional caregivers (*Continued*)
  nonverbal communication and,
    55–56
  resilience/absorbing suffering of,
    118–20
  "sharing the darkness" by, 122–23
  training/vocation of, 61
  a word to, 117–18
  zealots and, 22–23

Realists, 21
Reflective moments, 41
Relationships, suffering influence
  on, 105
Resilience
  of professional caregivers,
    118–20
  strong feeling/impulse
    management and, 119
Respect, 111–13
  in conversation, 111–12
Role changes
  due to life-threatening diagnosis,
    30
  due to treatment, 30–31

Self-examination, 66
Self-help books, 82–83
Self-reflection, 66

Sense of loss
  expression of, 29–30
  life aspects and, 29
  life span and, 30
  mortal time and, 29–31
Sense of urgency, from mortal time, 32
Sensitivity
  of death talk, 95
  people reading skills for, 108
  tentativeness and, 109
"Serenity Prayer"
  (Niebuhr, Reinhold), 111
"Sharing the darkness," 122–23
Shattered assumptions, 18–19
  adjustment after, 19
  by mortal time, 43–44
Sigler, Hollis, 39
Silence
  of caregivers, 69–70
  conversation and, 71
Spiritual belief/tradition
  assumptive work and, 18
  hope and, 45
  mortal time and, 16–17
Spontaneity
  without consideration, 83–84
  disciplined, 82–85
Stokes, Nina Ann, 66
Stone, Bob, 44

Stone Humphries, Jenny, 44
Suffering
    absorbance of, caregivers and,
        118–20
    companionship and, 104
    healing/helping in midst of,
        120
    honesty and, 73
    relationships influenced by, 105
Suicide, 34–35

Tactlessness, of professional
        caregivers, 26–27, 84–85
Thomas, W. I., 70
"tikkun olam", 123
Treatment
    mortal time during, 14
    receptionist/staff behavior during,
        101
    role changes due to, 30–31

Virtues needed in mortal time,
        106–17
    acceptance as, 110–11
    compassion as, 113 14
    courage as, 109–10

genuineness as, 106–7
    humor as, 114–16
    personal limitation awareness as,
        116–17
    presence as, 107–8
    respect as, 111–13
    sensitivity as, 108–9

"Well, you can't live forever," 81
"What can I say?", 70–72
Where the Buffaloes Roam (Stone,
        Bob/Stone Humphries,
        Jenny), 44
"Why me?", 19, 64
Williams, C. K., 123
Words
    can stay for a lifetime, 62
    humane use of, 81–82
    loss of, 71
    right, 72–73
World, benevolence/meaningfulness
        of, 19

Yood, James, 30

Zealots, 22–23

AUTHOR CONTACT INFORMATION

The authors welcome feedback and are available for speaking engagements. To contact them, write to Richard P. McQuellon, Ph.D., Wake Forest University Baptist Medical Center, Medical Center Blvd., Winston-Salem, NC 27157-1082, or email rmcquell@wfubmc.edu.